T0266928

YOGA INVERSIONS

YOGA INVERSIONS

Your Guide to Going Upside Down

KAT HEAGBERG REBAR

With photos by Andrea Killam
Foreword by Dianne Bondy

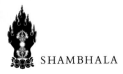

SHAMBHALA

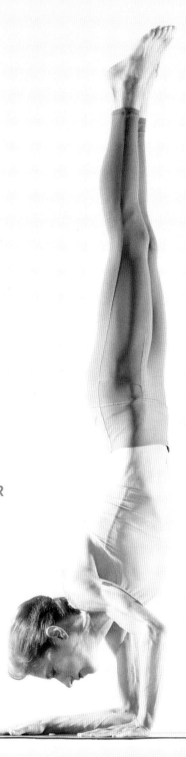

Shambhala Publications, Inc.
2129 13th Street
Boulder, Colorado 80302
www.shambhala.com

Note: The content of this book is not intended as medical advice. Please seek approval from your health-care practitioner before attempting any of the methods described here.

Cover Photos: Andrea Killam
Cover Design: Alex Hennig
Interior design: Laura Shaw Design

9 8 7 6 5 4 3 2 1

First Edition
Printed in Malaysia

Shambhala Publications makes every effort to print on acid-free, recycled paper.
Shambhala Publications is distributed worldwide by Penguin Random House, Inc., and its subsidiaries.

Library of Congress Cataloging-in-Publication Data

Names: Heagberg, Kat, author. | Killam, Andrea, photographer.
Title: Yoga inversions: your guide to going upside down / Kat Heagberg Rebar; with photos by Andrea Killam.
Description: First edition. | Boulder, Colorado: Shambhala Publications, Inc., [2023]
Identifiers: LCCN 2022035906 | ISBN 9781645471004 (trade paperback)
Subjects: LCSH: Yoga. | Hatha yoga.
Classification: LCC RA781.7 .H43 2023 | DDC 613.7/046— dc23/eng/20220912
LC record available at https://lccn.loc.gov/2022035906

Contents

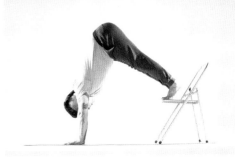

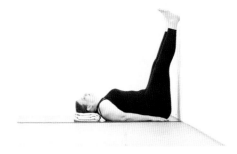
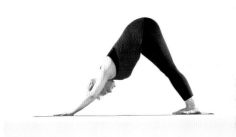
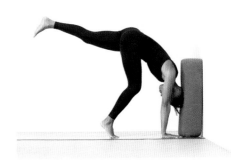
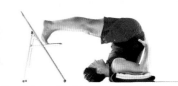

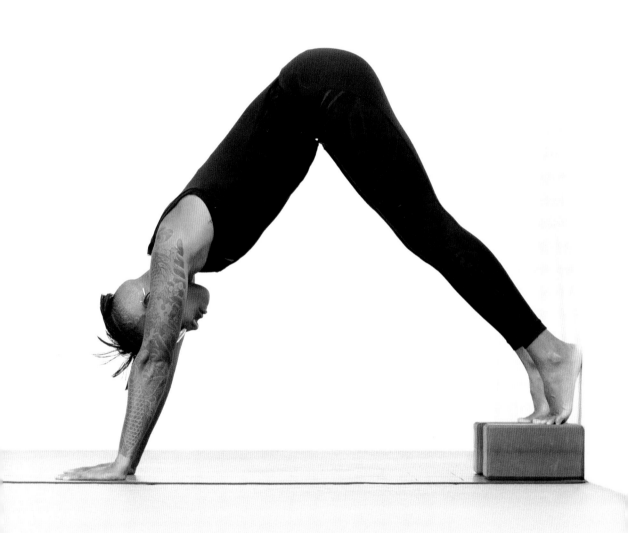

Foreword

I remember the very first time that I did yoga with my mom. I was three years old, and it was a fun way to move our bodies together. The time we spent together practicing asana was so special. I was one of three young children she had at that time, and she needed an outlet to find her center and allow for some quiet self-care time. My mother believed in intentional wellbeing well before it was widely practiced and commercialized.

Because of her example, I always thought of yoga as something I could do for myself without judgment about my ability or body. Until I stepped into a yoga studio. You see, I am a fat Black yoga practitioner, and during the 90s and early 2000s, we didn't see diversity in yoga spaces. I was often stared at or ignored as I struggled through complex asana variations. My home practice had always been about creating shapes that felt good and freeing to my body, but all of a sudden, a very flexible and highly annoyed yoga teacher was barking orders at me, and my body just couldn't do these poses. I was questioning what I understood yoga to be, and I felt a profound sense of shame about being "othered" in a space that was supposed to be rooted in union and nonviolence. I felt like I didn't belong, and I didn't return to a studio for a long time.

The next studio I practiced in was my own. I opened a yoga studio after that experience because I felt that I needed to create a space where people could practice yoga without being judged for what their bodies looked like and what they could or couldn't do. As a Black woman, I was no stranger to being overlooked or denied a seat at the table. I couldn't get hired as a yoga teacher, so I created my studio, where I could offer the kind of yoga that I myself wanted to explore: A practice that stems from the heart and soul of humanity. A practice grounded in understanding, equity, diversity, and community. All the studios in my town were about fancy poses, expensive clothes, and bendy young bodies. I needed more, so I created more.

I learned very early in life that the world isn't always going to be there for people who look like me or anyone who doesn't fit the mold of what society deems normal or acceptable. We have to create our own spaces where we feel seen and respected. (Long live Eastside Yoga Windsor community!)

Our community practiced together at a time when there were no books featuring people who looked like us doing yoga postures or accessible online platforms where we could do yoga without facing judgment and bias. I would have loved a book that showed me how to create asana shapes in my body. A book that evoked a sense of joy in moving around moving my body and exploring my breath in many different ways.

As a larger-bodied person, I always loved going upside down, proving to myself that I could create options that allowed me the same access to inversions as smaller people. I had to figure this out for myself. I am thrilled that Kat Heagberg Rebar, an incredible yoga educator, has created this book, *Yoga Inversions: Your Guide to Going Upside Down*, so that we have a guide that depicts a variety of bodies doing inversions.

Kat is an intuitive, thoughtful, and brilliant teacher. She shares her passion for going upside down with a sense of joy, rooted in experience and a commitment to equity. With this book, Kat has created a phenomenal resource that allows us to see bodies both like and unlike our own doing things we want to with step-by-step instructions to help us all find joy in the upside down.

Yoga Inversions is a beautifully inclusive book that illustrates that there is something for each of us to explore in our inversions practice.

No matter who you are—a yoga teacher, student, or general movement enthusiast—this book is for you. The skill and ease with which Kat will guide you through an inversion practice will give you the power to feel safe and strong in your body. You will gain personal insight into how this practice can be adapted to your body and all bodies.

Yoga Inversions lays the framework for finding your freedom in inversions. I encourage you to enjoy your practice with passion, compassion, and curiosity. Find the joy and playfulness of being upside down. You can do this. You are more powerful than you think!

—DIANNE BONDY

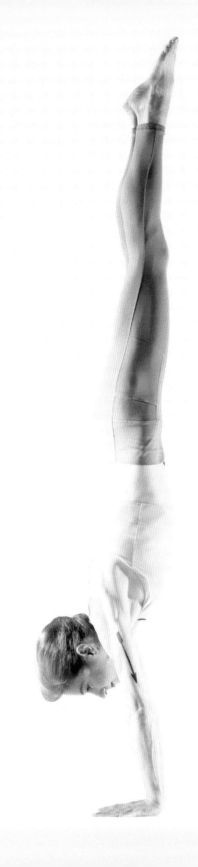

Preface

When I wrote *Yoga Where You Are: Customize Your Practice for Your Body and Your Life* with Dianne Bondy in 2020, my coauthor and I shared that we wrote the book that we—as longtime yoga students, teachers, and teacher trainers—wished existed: a comprehensive resource designed to grow with us; a book that didn't tell us what to do but gave us tools to figure it out on our own; hundreds of customizable variations demonstrated by folks who represent the yoga practitioners we know in real life and ideas and inspiration for building sequences that we could use for years to come. After receiving kind feedback from teachers all over the world, we quickly realized that we weren't the only ones who had been craving such a resource!

When it comes to this book, which takes a similar approach but focuses specifically on inversions, I can say that I wrote the book that I didn't even realize needed to exist but that, in retrospect, I certainly wish I'd had access to at the beginning of my inversion journey.

When my *Yoga Where You Are* editor Sarah Stanton asked if I'd be interested in writing another book and told me she had an idea, I was all ears. Anyone who knows me knows inversions—handstands in particular—are my *jam*. I'm constantly sharing tips and variations on Instagram. I regularly teach inversion-focused workshops and am often called in by colleagues to teach an inversion segment in yoga teacher trainings. My email avatar is a photo of me doing a handstand. At this point, there are probably more photos out there of me upside down than right side up! Or as my BFF Nam (who is also one of the models in this book) recently said, after I'd confessed to neglecting my Onewheel (electric skateboard) training for . . . several months . . . and didn't feel confident riding it through busy downtown traffic: "If you practiced your Onewheel half as much as you handstand, you'd be a pro by now." Noted (and I *promise* I'll get back to it soon, really!).

But back to the story. Sarah asked if I'd be interested in writing a book about how to do inversions, written in a similar customizable, inclusive, step-by-step way to *Yoga Where You Are*. She explained that there didn't seem to be any books out there that focused primarily on yoga inversions.

I was stunned! Surely there must be? But I couldn't find anything either. And I didn't take much (any) convincing to start writing exactly the kind of book I'd have wanted to have when I was learning inversions.

Though I was an active kid, I didn't grow up taking gymnastics, and I don't recall attempting a handstand at all until I was in college. And it would be another ten years before I tried doing forearm stands and handstands away from the wall.

It was through a combination of studying with a lot of different yoga teachers from a lot of different styles, scouring the internet for help and ideas, and a whole lot of trial and error that I learned to love inversions. And I'm delighted to share what I've learned with you here, in the pages of this book, so that you can save yourself some scouring and have a go-to resource to turn to for inspiration, encouragement, and helpful hints.

Whether you're brand-new to inversions, a seasoned handstander looking for new challenges, a yoga teacher seeking suggestions, or anywhere in between, I hope this book supports you wherever you are and wherever you're headed!

As with *Yoga Where You Are*, this book includes hundreds of customizable variations, demonstrated by real people representing a variety of bodies, abilities, ages, ethnicities, genders, and levels of experiences, all captured by the world's best yoga photographer, Andrea Killam.

My hope is that you use it to support and empower your practice and your life; that it meets you where you are and supports you as you change and grow.

—KAT HEAGBERG REBAR

YOGA INVERSIONS

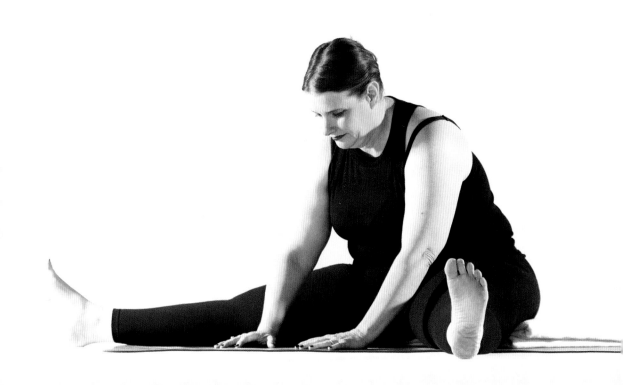

Introduction

Welcome! I can't wait to share the information in this book with you. That's because it's everything I wish I'd had at my fingertips when I started falling head-over-heels in love with yoga inversions—all the tips, hacks, and insights that I learned from skilled teachers and friends or figured out on my own through trial and error. (Trust me, there was a whole lot of error along the way!) I wrote this book to put everything I've learned in one place: to organize it, highlight it, and structure it in such a way that you can explore, learn, and develop your inversion practice while avoiding some of the frustrations and "stuck places" I faced along the way.

You can use this book in a variety of ways: Go straight to a pose you're interested in to learn tips and variations—you might find one in particular that you want to focus on or explore a variety of variations to see what works best for you.

You might also use or adapt some of the sample plans if they align with a goal of yours, such as learning a forearm balance or moving your handstand away from the wall. Like *Yoga Where You Are*, this book is designed to grow with you, and I offer plenty of options for gradually progressing your practice if and as you're ready to. Teachers can also find plenty of inspiration for their classes and for enhancing their own practice of inversions.

Each chapter explores a specific type of inversion (downward-facing dog and dolphin pose, handstand, forearm stand, headstand, and shoulderstand and plow) and includes general information about benefits and contraindications; preps and drills to help you build strength, enhance mobility, and hone key skills; dozens of customizable variations; handy tips and prop hacks; practice plans; and ways to incorporate inversions into a yoga practice.

Here are some specific ways that you can use it to meet and support you where you are right now:

IF YOU'RE NEW TO YOGA OR INVERSIONS AND WANT TO LEARN THEM FROM SCRATCH

Start with chapter 1 on page 6 to get a sense of what inversions are and how to approach them and to learn about some common misconceptions about them that you may encounter on your journey. Then I recommend heading over to chapter 2, which focuses on finding your own optimal downward-facing dog and dolphin pose variations. These asanas (poses) will be your foundation for other more complicated inversions, so by starting with that foundation, you're setting yourself up for success! From there, check out chapter 3 on handstand—in particular, the handstand preps and drills beginning on page 29 and the "walking into handstand" options on page 40 that will show you how to take the next steps (pun intended!) in turning your downward-facing dog into a handstand!

Even if you're learning to hop or jump up into a handstand *at* the wall (which I definitely recommend to start!), you can use the one-month "Take Your Handstand Off the Wall" plan on page 176 and simply substitute the five-minute handstand practice at the end of days two and three with any of the "walking into handstand" options on page 40. Or you can use the template in the appendix on page 188 to create your own custom plan, incorporating any of the drills, preps, and variations that you like! As you progress in your practice, select other handstand variations that you'd like to explore or check out some of the other chapters on forearm stand, headstand, and more.

If handstand is contraindicated for you or just not interesting to you, you could instead start by exploring the dolphin variations beginning on page 23 and then move right to chapter 4 on forearm stand. There too, explore the preps and drills (beginning on page 98) and then use or adapt the plan on page 182 that's designed to help you learn forearm stand.

If you're brand-new at this going-upside-down thing and looking for a more restorative inversion practice, check out the legs-up-the-wall variations on page 153 or the inverted action pose (viparita karani) variations on page 156. These poses are often gentle and simple enough to practice on their own (legs-up-the-wall variations can feel particularly wonderful after a long day of traveling or being on your feet), but you can also use the yoga-sequence template on page 195 in the appendix for ideas on how you might incorporate them into a complete yoga practice.

IF YOU HAVE A SPECIFIC INVERSION GOAL

Want to learn to balance on your forearms without flipping over? Ready to move your handstand away from the wall? Want to build strength and stability for a sustainable headstand? Or maybe you've been hopping into handstand for ages and are ready to embark on the "quest for the press" (pressing up into a handstand from a forward bend without using any momentum)?

Then I think you're going to love this book! In the process of writing it, I worked with a group of motivated pals (some of whom you'll see modeling in the pages of this book) and asked them the following questions:

- What's your inversion goal? (For example, learn to do a handstand, learn to do a handstand away from the wall, learn to do a forearm stand or headstand, learn to press into handstand, learn a pike press, and so forth.)

- What do you feel are your main obstacles in achieving this goal? (For example, lack of hip mobility, lack of upper-body strength/mobility, finding balance, overcoming fear, just getting up there!)

- Are there any poses or exercises you *don't* want to include? (These could be contraindications or just things you don't like doing. After all, you're much more likely to stick with something if you enjoy it!)

- How often do you want to practice? (Most folks preferred about three 30-minute practices a week, which is why that's the format you'll find in the goal-based plans in this book, but you can certainly practice more if you like, or shorten the practices to ten to twenty minutes on days where you don't have much time.)

From there I created custom plans for each person in this "beta group": Three days a week, thirty minutes, for one month. We checked in regularly and tweaked and adjusted the plans as needed to address any challenges that came up along the way. And though this beta group was fairly small, everyone who stuck with their one-month plan ended up achieving their goal! (In fact, Kyle, who you can get to know on page 201, set a goal of learning to do a middle-of-the-room handstand in one month, but he ended up meeting his goal in a week! So in his case, he created a new goal (achieving a handstand push-up).

The goal-based plans in this book, which you'll find at the end of the chapters on handstand, forearm stand, and headstand, were created based on these "sample plans." You can use them as is, you can tweak them to better fit your own needs and goals, or you can create a plan that's entirely your own, using the template on page 188 in appendix 1. You could start by asking yourself the same questions that I asked my friends when creating their plans, and you can incorporate any of the preps and drills in this book in order to address your own unique challenges. All the preps and drills include not only instructions on *how* to practice them (labeled "in practice") but also their purpose: *why* to practice them in order to learn and hone inversions (simply labeled "purpose"). This makes it easy for you to select those that match up with your own unique challenges.

IF YOU'RE LOOKING FOR WAYS TO INCORPORATE INVERSIONS INTO YOUR PERSONAL YOGA PRACTICE

Each chapter contains helpful suggestions for how and when to include the featured variations in practice, but you can also turn to the sample yoga-sequence blueprint on page 195 of appendix 2 to get ideas for where and how to place the featured inversions in a complete home yoga sequence.

IF YOU'RE A YOGA OR MOVEMENT TEACHER

Use the variations in this book as tools to help your students customize inversions so they leave your classes with a feeling of success and empowerment!

You can also use the sample sequence blueprint on page 195 as a framework for planning inversion-focused yoga classes. Or you might decide you'd like to teach a workshop on a particular inversion or goal, in which case you can explore the chapter focused on that inversion or skill for inspiration or use the goal-based template to create a custom one-month "plan" for your participants to walk away with! (One of my most popular workshops is a "Take Your Handstand Off the Wall" workshop, and participants love getting a copy of the plan on page 176 to keep their momentum going for learning and practice after the workshop is over.)

You can also use the goal-based plans in this book, or create your own using the goal template, in your work with private students and small groups.

And remember, though this book contains literally hundreds of customizable variations, *customizable* is the key word. I hope that you'll use the tools and tips here to support the real, actual people who walk into your classes: If a particular variation doesn't work, try something else! As my improv teacher always says, "Play to the top of your knowledge and experience." In the context of a yoga teacher's role, this means using the learned and lived knowledge that *you* have to create variations and preps of your own! These variations are here to inspire your creativity, not just to tell you "what to do."

IF YOU'RE A TEACHER TRAINER IN A 200-, 300-, OR 500-HOUR PROGRAM

I encourage you to use this book as part of your curriculum in order to show your participants a variety of ways that inversions can be learned and adapted. In particular, this book can be a key resource when you explore inversions as a pose category, sequencing, how to adapt asanas, advanced pose variations, and working with private clients. Though this book is intended as a resource for inversion enthusiasts of all levels, I wrote it specifically with teacher trainings in mind. As with *Yoga Where You Are*, I wanted to write the sort of book that I'd wished for, both as a participant in teacher trainings and later as a teacher who facilitated them: something that organized everything all in one place, that featured people who represented me and the folks who came to my classes, and that was easy to understand without being overly simplistic—a book that could travel along with me throughout my lifelong yoga journey!

BEFORE YOU BEGIN: PROPS AND SUPPLIES TO HAVE ON HAND

Some of the variations featured in this book use props. I consider myself a "prop minimalist." I love props, and I regularly use a variety of them in my own practice, but I tend to get overwhelmed with pose variations that require me to use a whole bunch at one time. And as a teacher, especially one who often teaches classes online, I also understand that most folks don't have an entire yoga-studio's worth of props on hand at home! That's why I try to keep it simple throughout this book. Most poses that incorporate props only use one or two props at a time. (Though there are some really cool ones that do use more; these are variations that I, the prop minimalist, find so helpful and interesting that I just couldn't resist including them!) The props featured in this book include:

- An open wall space
- Yoga blocks
- A yoga strap (a dog leash, bathrobe tie, necktie, long towel, or belt can serve as an easy substitute)
- A yoga chair or folding chair
- A bolster (a firm cushion or a thickly folded or rolled firm blanket can often be a good substitution)
- Blankets
- A sandbag (a bag of rice or beans, or even a folded blanket, can serve as an easy swap)
- A yoga mat (In some places you'll see this referred to as a "sticky mat," which means that you'll want to use a mat with good "grip." This is pretty much the case for any mat that's intended for yoga practice. I recommend avoiding "squishier" mats, like gym mats.)

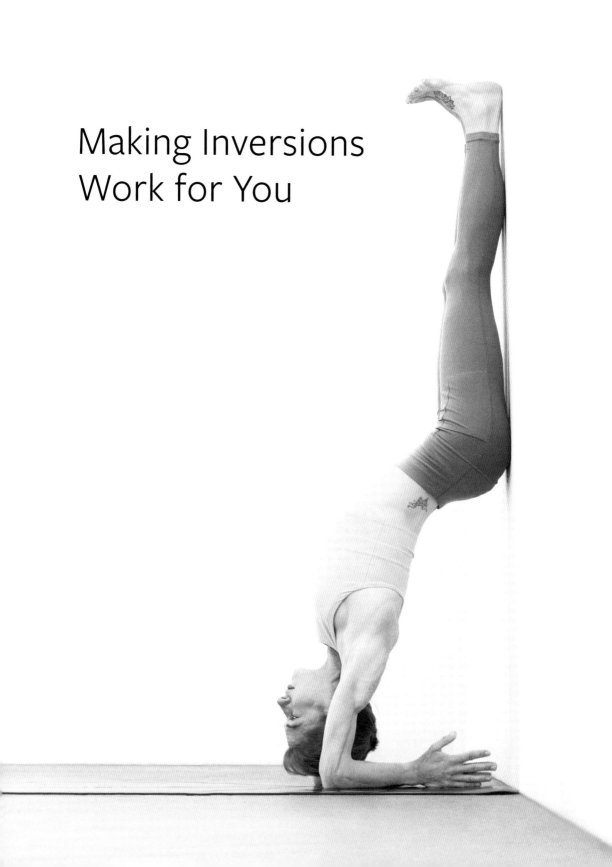

Making Inversions Work for You

What are inversions? As seems to be the case with anything in our wild, wonderful, yet still very imperfect and often confusing modern yoga world, different yoga teachers have different opinions on what constitutes an inversion.

Some say an inversion is any pose where your head is below your heart (this is also a common definition used in other movement modalities). By this definition, standing forward bends and poses such as downward-facing dog and dolphin (see chapter 2) count as inversions; however, many yoga teachers don't treat these poses as such when planning, theming, and sequencing their classes.

Others will say that inversions are poses where your legs are up in the air, reversing the effects of gravity and aiding in circulation. This definition includes poses like legs up the wall (page 153), where your head doesn't necessarily drop below the level of your heart.

Then there are those whose definition includes both requirements—head below heart, legs in the air—in order for a pose to "count" as an inversion.

And yet that still doesn't do it for others: Some teachers and styles of yoga require you to hold a pose for a long period of time, often at least a minute or more, for it to be categorized as an inversion. Adherents to this definition argue that it takes that long to truly experience the benefits of inverting. According to this school of thought, for the majority of us, more "active" inversions—those that typically require more of a strength or balance challenge like handstands and forearm stands—are out. According to these teachers and styles, those poses are usually categorized as arm balances or hand balances but not inversions.

I, for one, am not particularly invested in arguing semantics in order to sway anyone's opinion here. I have learned from many skilled yoga and movement teachers who hold a variety of opinions on this matter, but for the purpose of this book, I'm choosing to take the most inclusive approach possible, including all of the aforementioned poses and more.

That's because these poses share many of the same benefits and similar characteristics, which makes them complement one another well. For example, working with downward-facing dog builds essential skills and strength for handstand, and for most versions of handstand in yoga, you'll enter via downward-facing dog. So in this context, diving into both makes a lot of sense.

This also gives us a lot more options to work with—more variations for teachers reading this to share with students in order to create classes that are customizable, inclusive, and empowering for everyone who shows up.

And I firmly believe that teaching yoga asanas should be about giving folks the tools to customize any given shape or movement for their unique bodies in order to support their unique needs and goals. Yoga is not about "fixing" ourselves or anyone else or causing discomfort by trying to make our bodies fit some "ideal" version of an asana. In other words, I'm all about doing yoga to enhance your life, not making your whole life about doing yoga poses for their own sake.

That's part of what makes yoga *yoga*. It's not about what the poses look like; it's about something deeper. Something better.

THE HISTORY AND SIGNIFICANCE OF INVERSIONS IN YOGA

Yoga has a rich history, and in our book *Yoga Where You Are*, Dianne Bondy and I explore this in more detail—including yoga's roots and origins in India and Kemetic yoga practices from the continent of Africa.

While this book is primarily a practice and teaching companion focused on asanas, it's always important to acknowledge the origins of yoga practice, which is and has long been sacred to many people. This doesn't mean you have to "believe in" any particular religion or the supernatural (I myself do not). But we can still give credit where credit is due. We can pay homage to the culture and context in which yoga originated and acknowledge that for many people in this world, yoga is more than exercise.

To learn more about honoring and acknowledging yoga's roots, I highly recommend Susanna Barkataki's book *Embrace Yoga's Roots: Courageous Ways to Deepen Your Yoga Practice*. This book is a must-read for anyone who teaches yoga today, particularly those of us who benefit from white privilege.

And if you're a yoga-history geek like me, I recommend checking out Richard Rosen's *Original Yoga: Rediscovering Traditional Practices of Hatha Yoga*. This is a longtime favorite of mine that I recommend to students in all my teacher trainings to help provide clarity and context about key yoga texts that include descriptions of asanas and other physical practices. (A plea to my fellow teacher trainers: The Yoga Sutra and the Bhagavad Gita are no doubt rich, fascinating, and important, but there are other ancient yoga works worth reading too!) In *Original Yoga*, Rosen looks at three historical hatha yoga texts: the *Hatha Yoga Pradipika*, the *Gheranda Samhita*, and the *Shiva Samhita*, explaining their context and exploring ways in which the practices in these books could be adapted to be more relevant to our lives today.

These three ancient practice manuals discuss *pranayama* (breathwork intended to control or expand *prana*, or "life force"), meditation, *bandhas* ("locks" intended to regulate and influence the movement of prana), *mudras* (sacred gestures), *kriyas* (cleansing practices), and asanas—including some inversions and mudras that can be adapted and explored within the context of inversions.

And, of course, if we look at the modern history of yoga in the twentieth century, we can clearly see that inversions were highlighted prominently in styles such as Ashtanga yoga and Iyengar yoga. Though by no means the only players in modern postural yoga, these two schools strongly influenced the way that we view, practice, teach, and depict yoga today.

Though thanks in part to the influence of the aforementioned styles, we tend to focus more on the physical, health-related benefits of inversions nowadays. But many folks today still use inversions for spiritual purposes, including as tools to explore and influence the subtle body (which includes, among other things, prana, *nadis*—the channels that prana is said to move through—and chakras—the energetic "hubs" where many nadis intersect). For example, I once learned a practice from yoga teacher Sandra Anderson, which used inversions such as inverted action pose, shoulderstand, plow, and headstand to "enliven and activate" *udana vayu*, which is the upward flow of prana.

In a Yoga International article[*] on this topic she explains, "Since udana is an ascending force, poses that . . . turn the body upside down are especially beneficial for activating udana." And again, it's totally fine if this doesn't resonate with you. You don't have to believe in the subtle body, and you don't have to practice in this way, but I do think it's both respectful to yoga's roots and provides useful context to acknowledge it.

---

[*] Sandra Anderson, "The 5 Prana Vayus in Yoga: Udana," Yoga International, May 24, 2013, https://yogainternational.com/article/view/the-5-prana-vayus-in-yoga-udana.

MYTHS ABOUT INVERSIONS

There are many misconceptions that persist in the yoga world, and for one reason or another, a whole lot of them relate to inversions. Let's unpack a few here.

Inversions are only for "advanced" yoga practitioners.

Nope. While there are certainly inversions that require a lot of preparation and practice, there are others that are suitable for beginners, and there are also ways to regress more complicated poses. Note: *Regress* is the movement-science term for going back a few steps and simplifying a pose or movement in order to prepare for it, hone it, or isolate a particular skill. Its companion term, *progress*, refers to adding to or changing elements of a movement in order to increase challenge. Both terms are value neutral (a progression is not superior to a regression), and yoga and movement practitioners of all levels use these strategies to support their goals and intentions.

It's also wise for teachers to remember that just because someone is a beginner in yoga doesn't mean that they're a beginner to all forms of movement; *advanced* and *beginner* are relative terms. A gymnast who has done handstand presses for years could come to a yoga class for the very first time and be just fine to try one, and someone with an intricate knowledge of yoga who has been practicing every day for decades may find that a restorative legs-up-the-wall pose is their go-to inversion of choice.

If inversions are contraindicated for you, this book has nothing to offer you.

Okay, so this myth is unique to this book, but I think it's important to address. My intention in writing this book is to offer as many customizable options and tools as possible so that anyone who wants to can experience the benefits of inversions, even if they are unable to literally go upside down.

This goal became extra clear when I asked my cousin Sarah (who you'll soon meet in the pages that follow) if she'd like to model for my upcoming yoga book. Sarah is not a big yoga fan, but she's no stranger to movement and athleticism—she does all sorts of dance and even convinced me to attend my first Bollywood aerobics class (a high recommend, by the way). She attends boot-camp classes on the regular, hikes every day—you get the idea. I wanted to feature her for this reason: to represent folks like her who weren't that into yoga but were still super active and might like to explore inversions.

About a week before our photo shoot, I mentioned that the book was about inversions specifically and asked Sarah what poses she was most comfortable modeling. That's when she said, "Oh, inversions are contraindicated for me; is this going to be okay?"

I thought about it for a moment and was like, "Yes, of course!" Because there are plenty of ways to get the benefits of inversions and work with the actions they require without actually flipping upside down, and in this book I will show you how.

In Sarah's case, forward bends and mild inversions like downward-facing dog variations are fine for her, but I also include poses that keep your head at or above the level of your heart and/or both of your feet on the ground.

People who menstruate should always avoid inversions during "that time of the month."

This is one that just won't quit. No one has to do *any* pose during menstruation or any other time if they don't want to, for any reason. If inverting on your period doesn't feel good for you, or if you just don't feel like it, then absolutely, don't do it! But if you *do* feel like inverting when you have your period, you'll probably be just fine. As a person who has experienced menstruation, I have never felt the need to quell my inversions. In fact, I often found that going upside down helped to relieve some of the cramping and digestive discomfort I would sometimes get.

And you might say, "Okay, Kat, so you felt good, but is it *safe*?" As far as I have found reviewing relevant research studies, and according to the midwives and ob-gyns I've spoken to, there is no reason why it's unsafe for the average menstruating human to do an inversion while menstruating. When I was the editor in chief at Yoga International, I edited and fact-checked a detailed article on this topic, and in the process I learned quite a bit! For example, folks with periods and their yoga teachers are still often told that inverting can cause retrograde menstruation, leading to endometriosis, but we know now that there isn't good evidence to support that claim. As the author Leah Sugerman writes,

> It was previously believed that inverting during one's period would lead to retrograde menstruation, in which blood would flow in the opposite direction through the fallopian tubes and result in the presence of uterine tissue in the pelvic cavity—tissue that would embed itself there and lead to endometriosis. More is now known about endometriosis, and its relationship to retrograde menstruation is not as clear-cut as once believed.

First of all, it seems the majority of [menstruating people] experience some degree of retrograde menstruation (90% in one study), while only about 10% develop endometriosis. The current view is that (at least in the absence of "overwhelming amounts of endometrial cells") endometriosis occurs when there is an impaired immune response, and/or when the endometrial cells themselves are "abnormal"—i.e., in secreting higher than usual levels of inflammatory cytokines, which make them more likely to embed and grow outside the uterus. In most people who experience what we might call a "normal" amount of retrograde menstruation each month, the immune system deals well with any stray uterine cells in the pelvic cavity, so that the majority of us will never develop endometriosis.

Further, according to at least one expert, you needn't worry that inversions will increase retrograde menstruation (and consequently, your chances of developing endometriosis), because uterine contractions, rather than your orientation to the ground, are responsible for the flow of menstrual blood. That would explain why we can menstruate when floating in space in the same way we do when standing upright on the ground.[*]

So why does this myth persist? For one, due to a variety of societal factors and sex and gender biases, a lot of us don't know as much as we should about how menstruation works. And on an "intuitive" level, it does kind of make sense: If we go upside down, won't that "reverse the flow," and wouldn't that be bad, because menstrual fluid is supposed to flow down and out? As Sugerman explains, that's not exactly how that works, but it's understandable to come to that conclusion if you haven't learned otherwise.

Plus, remember, when it comes to yoga, it's also not all about physiology. Some teachers say that from a pranic ("energetic" or subtle-body-related) point of view, inverting during menstruation disrupts *apana*, the downward flow of prana. If this is relevant to your beliefs and practice, it's a valid reason to skip inversions (as is *any* reason; when it comes to your body, you get to decide). But it doesn't make inverting unsafe. And as a yoga teacher, I don't think it's a good reason for me to impose a restriction on someone else or to make anyone else's period any of my business.

Finally, the obvious reason this myth seems to persist: sex and gender bias specifically in the yoga world. Of course, these problems exist outside of yoga, but I'm still regularly disappointed when I realize how deeply embedded they are in yoga,

* Leah Sugerman, "Is It Safe to Practice Inversions during Menstruation?" Yoga International, June 15, 2017, https://yogainternational.com/article/view/is-it-safe-to-practice-inversions-during-menstruation1.

and how often yoga philosophy and tradition is misappropriated in order to enforce gender binaries and sexism. When I was preparing to write this section of the book, I spoke to the yoga researcher and author Dr. Steffany Moonaz, who is currently writing about the ways in which sexism and gender bias influence yoga research, and what she shared with me was pretty shocking. For example, I learned that menstruating people are often precluded from participating in yoga studies, many of which don't involve inverting at all but only gentle asanas and breathing practices. That's a huge chunk of the population that's left out, affecting the methodology of the studies and influencing the researchers' findings. It's these same outdated attitudes that keep people from unnecessarily avoiding movements that they love and that might actually help them feel *better* during their periods when they don't actually need to avoid them.

People who are pregnant should not ever do any inversions.

Sensing a trend here? I started teaching yoga when I was very young, and as a new teacher, not even old enough to order myself a post-class cocktail if I'd wanted to, I was nervous when a pregnant person came to class. I didn't know anything about pregnancy, and I was afraid I would teach something that could harm them or cause pregnancy complications. Being the type A, oldest child, Virgo, overachiever that I am, I immediately signed up for a weekend prenatal yoga training. Followed by a full prenatal teacher training. Followed by an entire yearlong doula program at a midwifery college (yes, really). And finally, I took some biology classes in a medical program. Through all of that, plus getting to an age where a lot of my friends were getting pregnant, I learned that pregnant people are much less fragile than I thought.

That doesn't mean you should *start* doing challenging inversions like handstands and headstands for the first time if you're pregnant. The general recommendation from health-care providers seems to be that unless your provider says otherwise, it's okay to continue the activities you did before pregnancy as long as they still feel good. That means if you enjoyed inversions before, you can likely continue to enjoy them as long as they're still enjoyable.

That said, every body, pregnancy, and situation is different; if you're pregnant, ask your doctor or midwife if inversions are okay for you, and be sure to mention what kind of inversions you're doing—there's a big difference between a legs-up-the-wall pose and a five-minute shoulderstand!

To err on the side of caution, there are also teachers, coaches, and medical professionals who recommend avoiding long holds in challenging inversions during pregnancy: Coming into a handstand at the wall for a couple of seconds if you're experienced and feel stable and confident? Sure. But maybe skip the five-minute shoulderstand for now.

Inversions can cure diabetes, regulate your metabolism, rid you of IBS, dispel all your "toxins" (whatever that means), heal depression and anxiety, [insert other "too good to be true" claims here] . . .

Inversions can feel great, and they do have benefits, but they're not cure-alls and they're not magic. If a claim sounds too good to be true, it probably is.

There is an ideal or best or "fullest expression" of every inversion.

If I can convince you of anything with this book, I hope it's that there is no one "right" way to do any yoga pose. The right version is the version that's right for you, right now. And *the* fullest expression is *your* fullest expression: the one that best serves your needs and goals today.

Every inversion is for every body.

Also false. While it's important for yoga teachers to be able to adapt their classes and the asanas they teach to best serve the people who show up, that doesn't mean that every pose or variation is for everyone. There are plenty of variations that aren't ideal for me, including some of the ones in this book, which is why you'll see a variety of different bodies represented.

As you read this book, I encourage you to take what works for you, change and adapt it if and as needed, and leave behind anything that isn't relevant or helpful for your life and practice.

Props are only used to make inversions easier.

Anyone who claims this is true has never attempted a handstand press with blocks under their hands (that makes it a lot harder, FYI). Props are tools we can use to regress a pose, progress a pose, or hone a specific action. As far as difficulty goes, they're a neutral element you can use in a variety of ways to create the most effective practice for you.

INVERSIONS AND ACCESSIBILITY

Though not every pose or variation is appropriate or ideal for everyone, I hope that this book in some way helps to make inversions more accessible. To show you that just because you didn't learn to handstand as a kid—which, by the way, I didn't—it doesn't mean you can't learn one as an adult if you want to. And that inversions can be customized, adapted, remixed, and tweaked to work for a variety of bodies, ages, levels, and abilities.

A note for teachers: In particular, I urge yoga teachers to remember that accessibility is more than just adapting poses—it's about the language that we use. It's about making our yoga spaces truly welcoming for people from marginalized communities. It's about not just acknowledging but *celebrating* body diversity, ethnic diversity, gender diversity, age diversity, neurodiversity, and more. Jivana Heyman and the Accessible Yoga community are doing incredible work in these areas and have some amazing resources for us. I encourage you, my colleagues, to visit accessibleyoga.org to see for yourself what they have to offer.

Ready to go upside down?

Downward-Facing Dog
(Adho Mukha Svanasana)
+ Dolphin Pose

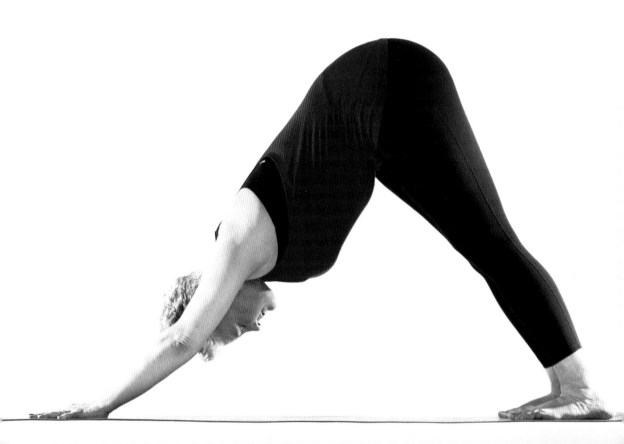

Downward-facing dog is the foundation for handstand. It can also be an inversion in its own right because in many of its variations (including the "classic" variation), your head is below your heart.

If you're working toward handstand, it's the perfect place to play with your hand and arm positions and to find what works best for you. It's also a very common entry point for hopping or jumping into handstand.

Similarly, dolphin pose is essentially downward-facing dog on your forearms, and it's a fabulous alternative to or preparation for forearm stand.

BENEFITS

These poses are also excellent "reset" poses to practice between asymmetrical asanas and vinyasa flows (a series of poses linked together). When practiced regularly, they can help build upper-body strength, increase flexibility in your hamstrings and calves, and help you to find a long, neutral spine position, which can be helpful in your yoga and movement practices overall.

GENERAL CONTRAINDICATIONS

Wrist, shoulder, and spinal injuries or recent surgeries, and untreated high blood pressure are considered contraindicated for downward-facing dog. Contraindications for dolphin are similar, though those with wrist issues may find it to be a fine alternative. If you're unsure if a pose is right for you, check with your doctor or other qualified medical professional such as a physical or occupational therapist.

Downward-Facing Dog with Hands on the Wall

Downward-facing dog with hands on the wall is a great variation to work with if you'd like to bear less weight through your hands, arms, and shoulders or if, like Sarah, who is demonstrating the "hands above shoulders" version below, inversions (i.e., "head below heart") are contraindicated for you but you still want to experience many of the benefits of downward-facing dog.

    If you're a yoga teacher, this variation also makes a great transition pose for at-the-wall flows. (I particularly like to include this one in my prenatal classes!)

Hands-Above-Shoulders Version

Place your hands on the wall with your arms straight and your hands about shoulder-width apart, with your wrist creases making a straight line and your fingers spread a comfortable distance apart. (You can also turn your hands in or out a little more if that feels better for you; experiment and see what works best!)

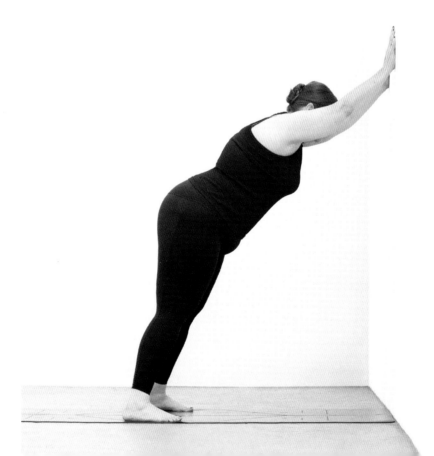

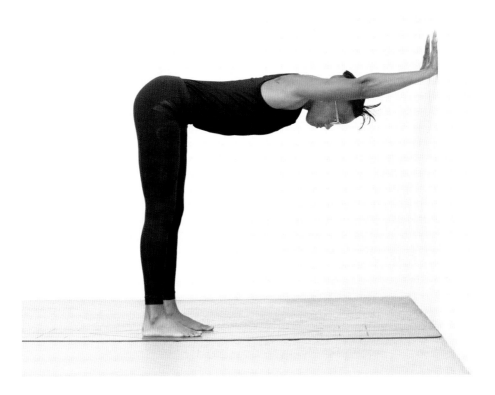

L-Shape Version

If you'd like to come into more of an L shape at the wall (as Shanté is demonstrating here), your wrist creases will be a little below shoulder height. (You can experiment with both and see what feels best for you! The V-shape variation is more similar in shape to a classic downward-facing dog, and the L-shape version is more of a hand-stand prep/first step!)

To make more of a V shape like Sarah (on page 18), have your hands at or slightly above shoulder height. Walk your feet back, bringing your heels beneath your hips. Try to keep your ears in line with your upper arms (avoid dropping your head or lifting your chin, and reach forward through your crown). Roll your inner upper arms upward.

Try to find as much length through your spine as you can. (Hint: bending your knees can help!)

Press your hands into the wall and reach back through your hips.

Stay for three to five breaths, then walk your feet toward the wall and your hands up the wall to come out, releasing your arms alongside you to finish.

Downward-Facing Dog with Hands on a Chair

Like downward-facing dog at the wall, these versions are fabulous for folks who want a less weight-bearing downward-facing dog option, and they're fun to include in chair-yoga flows that include standing options.

Tip: To keep your chair from sliding, place all four chair legs on a yoga mat as Sarah and I have done in the photos.

Hands-on-Chairback Version

If you want or need to avoid dropping your head below your heart (or you just prefer a little more height for your chair dog), try this version, with your hands holding the very top of the chair.

You can do this with the chair seat facing toward you (as Sarah is demonstrating in the photo) or away from you, depending on the type of chair you use and the pose you may wish to come into next if you're incorporating this into a chair-yoga flow.

————

Hold on to the top of the chair with both hands, then walk your feet back behind you, lengthening your arms and spine to find downward-facing dog.

Try to align the back of your head with the back of your pelvis. Bend your knees if that helps you to find even more length through your spine. If you can keep your spine long, experiment with straightening your legs a bit to get more of a stretch through the backs of your legs.

Stay for three to five breaths, then walk your feet back toward the chair to come out of the pose.

Hands-on-Chair-Seat Version

This version mimics the more "traditional" downward-dog shape where your spine is at a diagonal and your head is below your heart.

————

Stand facing the chair seat and place your hands on it. (I like to wrap my fingers around the edge of the seat, which feels extra stable and keeps my wrists in a more neutral position.) Walk your feet back behind you, lengthening your arms and your spine to find downward-facing dog. Keep your head in line with your spine and your neck long on all sides. You can bend your knees if you like or play with straightening your legs. Rotate your upper arms in toward your ears to release tension through your neck.

Stay for three to five breaths, then walk your feet toward the chair seat to come out.

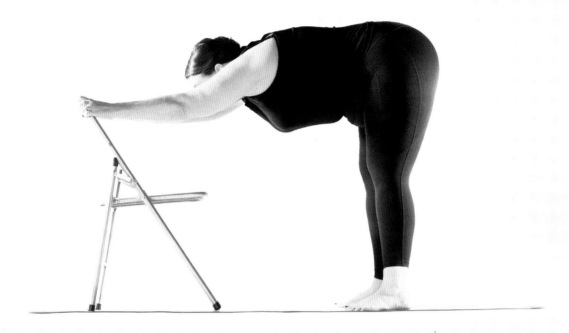

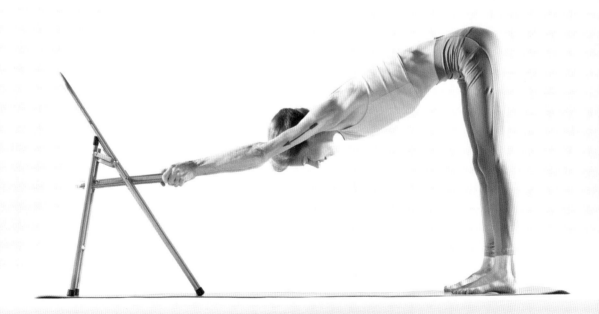

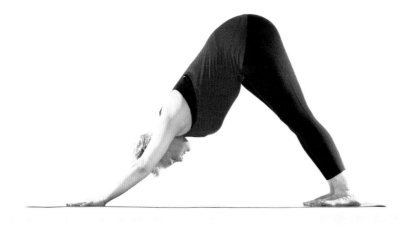

Downward-Facing Dog on the Mat

Start on hands and knees with toes tucked under, knees below hips, and hands below shoulders. From there, walk your hands one handprint forward so they're in front of your shoulders.

Begin with your hands shoulder-width apart, the creases of your wrists parallel with the top edge of your mat, and your fingers a comfortable distance apart. If this doesn't feel great, experiment with bringing your hands wider than shoulder-width and/or turning your hands out or in a little to see what feels best in your body.

Inhale here, then on an exhale, lift your knees and press your hips up and back to come into downward-facing dog.

Start with knees bent. Press your hands into the floor and your thighs back behind you to begin to straighten your legs a little or a lot (as Peggy is in the photo). If your back starts to round as you do this, that's a sign to bend your knees a little more.

Soften your jaw and gaze back toward your feet, keeping your neck long on all sides. Roll your inner upper arms up toward the sky to release tension in your neck.

Stay for three to five breaths, then lower your knees to the floor to come out.

Prop Suggestions to Customize Your Downward-Facing Dog

- If you'd like to find a downward-facing dog that's more spacious (which can be helpful if you're stepping forward into a lunge from downward-facing dog) and take a little bit of pressure out of your hands and wrists, try placing your hands on blocks, wrapping your fingers around the edges to really "get a grip."

- If your calves feel tight, it might feel nice to support your heels on a rolled-up yoga mat or blanket.

- For a more restorative variation, try resting your forehead on a block.

For dolphin, begin on forearms and knees with your elbows right under your shoulders. You can keep your forearms parallel to each other, as Kyle is demonstrating in the second photo, or bring your palms together, as Nam is demonstrating in the first photo. (You can have your hands in prayer, like Nam, or interlace your fingers. If you interlace, be sure to tuck in your bottom pinky to avoid crushing it.) Hands together can help to keep your elbows from splaying and is a really nice option if your shoulders feel tight.

If your forearms are parallel, try turning your hands out a bit, which may help to prevent your elbows from splaying in this position.

Next, tuck your toes under and lift your knees away from the floor to come into dolphin.

Keep your head in line with your spine, and lengthen through your spine as much as possible. (As with downward-facing dog, bending your knees can help.)

Stay for three to five breaths, then lower your knees to release.

Dolphin with Hands Together

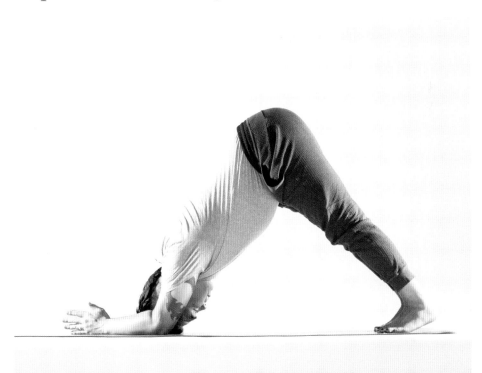

Dolphin with Forearms Parallel, Palms Down

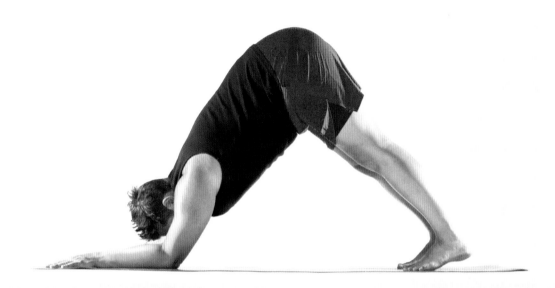

Other Hand and Arm Options

- If you're working toward parallel forearms but your elbows keep splaying apart, try holding a yoga block between your hands, gripping the sides with your fingers and thumbs.

- You can also loop a yoga strap around your upper arms and press out against the strap to keep elbows from splaying (page 113).

- To make dolphin more similar to downward-facing dog in shape and height while still going easy on your wrists, try elevating your forearms with blocks.

- For an added challenge that will increase the external rotation required in your upper arms and shoulders (which can be helpful when preparing for backbendy inversions such as hollowback forearm stand on page 114), try practicing dolphin with parallel forearms and your palms facing *up* instead of down. (You can see me demonstrating this in forearm stand on page 112.)

Handstand
(Adho Mukha Vrksasana)

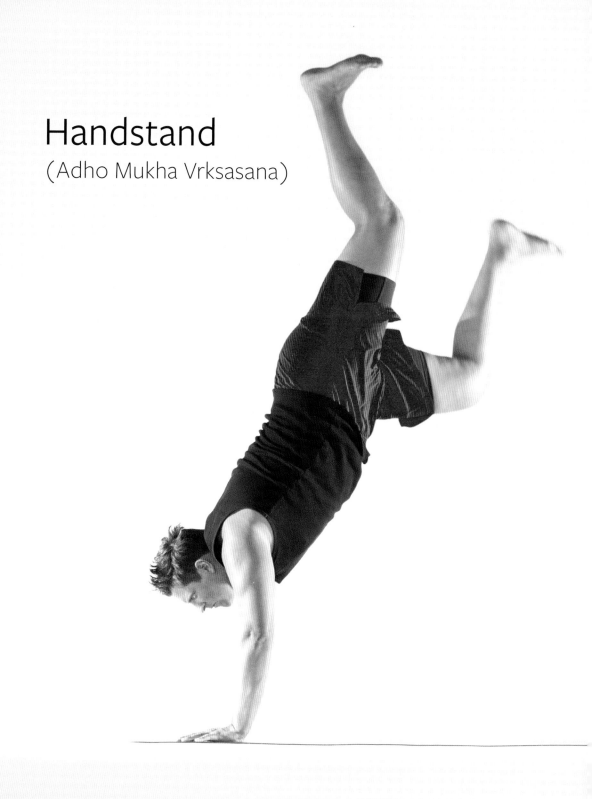

Handstand is not only my favorite inversion, it's also my favorite yoga pose, which isn't any surprise to folks who know me today. But it wasn't always that way.

I remember trying my first-ever handstand as a college freshman. I was practicing along to a yoga DVD, and the teacher presented the option of handstanding at the wall. I decided to give it a whirl, and I ended up loudly and inelegantly slamming my legs against the hall closet doors (the only empty wall space I could find). It wasn't graceful, but I got up there! And so it continued for the next several years. I enjoyed practicing handstands at the wall in yoga class, and over time my transitions became a little more graceful. But I never thought I could handstand away from the wall. I figured that since I didn't grow up as a gymnast, it just wasn't in the cards for me.

But after watching fellow practitioners hop, jump, or even press (!) into handstands in the middle of the room, I began to wonder if maybe it could be possible for me too. After all, these people weren't gymnasts or contortionists; they were just regular folks in my neighborhood. So I started practicing more regularly, gradually moving away from the wall a little more each day. (And, okay, falling over a few times too!)

Learning how to handstand, I've decided, is a lot like falling in love: it happens over time, and then all at once! Once I felt confident hopping into handstand in the middle of the room, I figured out how to jump off of two feet, and then how to press up without momentum. The key to taking my handstands off the wall and learning new variations and transitions, it turned out, was actually trying them. (Who knew!) Of course, the skills I honed with my wall handstands and other aspects of my yoga practice helped a lot.

In this chapter, I'm going to share with you some preps, drills, and variations that I've found particularly helpful over the years, both for myself and for working with students. Whether you want to learn to handstand at the wall for the first time, take your handstand away from the wall, or finesse your handstand press, there's something here for you!

BENEFITS OF HANDSTAND: WHY LEARN HANDSTAND BEFORE HEADSTAND OR SHOULDERSTAND?

Handstand requires—and thus builds—wrist, arm, shoulder, and core strength. I also find it can be a great way to lift my mood when I need a boost, and the process of learning, honing, and progressing it is a great confidence builder!

You might wonder why handstand appears so early in this book—before headstand and shoulderstand in particular, which are often easier for a lot of folks to get into. There are different schools of thought on this—and if you have zero interest in handstanding, you can certainly skip this chapter—but I generally adhere to the school of thought that exploring handstand and/or forearm balance first can be beneficial overall. That's because while these poses can be more challenging to learn initially, they're generally considered less "risky" than headstand and shoulderstand because you're not bearing weight through your head and/or neck. On a related note, the skills and strength you develop learning how to do handstand and forearm balance will help you to practice headstand and shoulderstand more sustainably and confidently.

This doesn't mean that you have to execute a "perfect" middle-of-the-room handstand or forearm stand before you ever attempt headstand or shoulderstand, but the preps, drills, and variations you explore while learning to balance on your hands and forearms can benefit your inversion practice overall.

You'll also notice that this chapter is longer than the others, and that's not just because handstand is my favorite pose. It's because many of the skills and strategies in this chapter can be adapted to the other inversions in this book, and I will refer back to them from time to time when I feel they might be useful. For example, pressing into a handstand is similar to the strategies you'll use to come into a headstand with control. And hopping into handstand is similar to hopping into forearm stand.

GENERAL CONTRAINDICATIONS

High blood pressure, glaucoma, and any condition where you need to avoid increased eye pressure; and wrist, shoulder, or spinal injuries or recent surgeries are considered contraindicated for handstand. If you're unsure whether handstand or any pose or variation in this book is a good idea for you, check with a licensed, credible medical provider before trying it.

Mountain Climbers

Purpose: To practice shifting your shoulders forward over your wrists and shifting weight into your fingertips, which is helpful for handstands in general and especially helpful if you're working toward press-handstand variations (page 54).

In Practice: From plank, draw one knee into your chest at a time, keeping your movement light and bouncy. To up the intensity, "jump switch" from one side to the other, as though you're running in place in plank. Continue for twenty to thirty seconds, rest for ten seconds, and repeat two to three more times if you like.

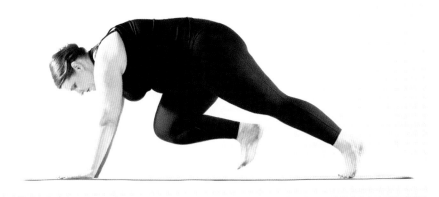

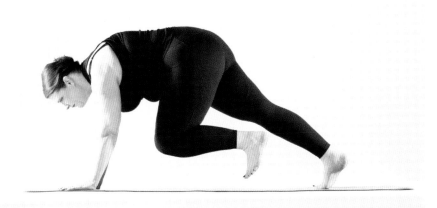

Yoga Burpees

Purpose: To mobilize your hips and develop skills for jumping into handstand.

In Practice: Begin in a high or low squat at the top of your mat with knees and toes pointing in the same direction. Then plant your hands in front of your feet (you'll need to lift your hips if you're in a low squat) and step or jump to a bent-knee downward-facing dog. Then step or jump forward back to your squat, bringing your hands to your heart, if you like, before planting them on the ground again to repeat. Do this for twenty to thirty seconds, rest for ten seconds, then repeat two to three more rounds if you like.

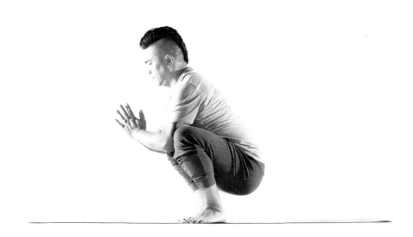

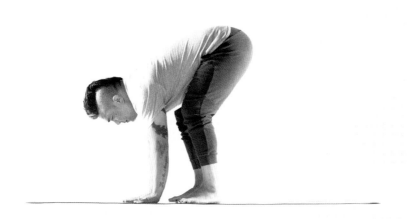

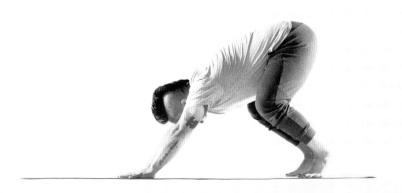

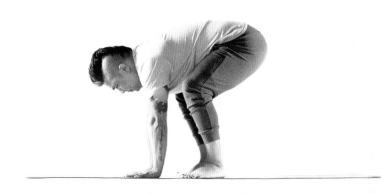

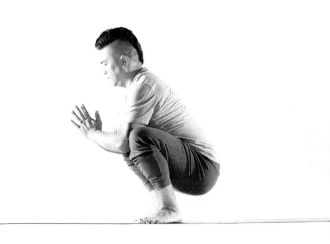

Side-to-Side Downward-Facing-Dog Jumps

Purpose: To develop skills for jumping into handstand and to work toward getting your hips up over your shoulders.

In Practice: From a bent-knee downward-facing dog, jump your feet to the left side of your mat, then the right, landing with your knees bent each time. To lower the intensity, step instead of jump.

Do this for twenty to thirty seconds, rest for ten seconds, then repeat two or three more rounds if you like.

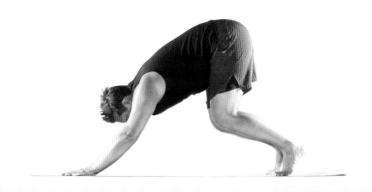

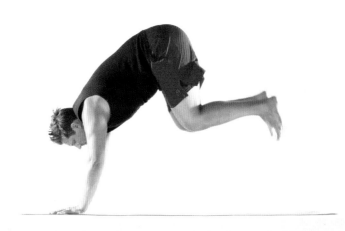

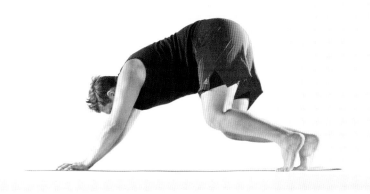

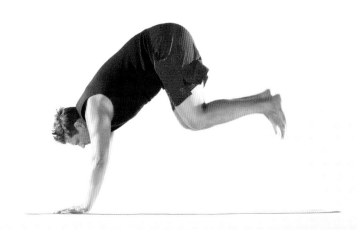

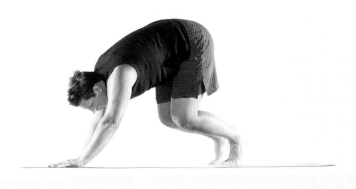

Lizard-Lunge Switches

Purpose: To mobilize your hips. (This can make hopping up into handstand a lot easier!)

In Practice: Begin in a wide lunge with your left foot forward and your hands inside your left foot—palms on the ground, or on fingertips, or with palms/fingertips on blocks, depending on what feels best. Aim to point your front knee and toes in the same direction. Inhale to prepare, then as you exhale, "jump switch" your legs so that your right leg is forward.

You can also "step switch" instead of jumping: With your left foot forward, rock back onto your left heel, lifting the sole of your left foot to build momentum, then step your right foot forward, outside of your right hand, and your left foot back to come into lizard lunge on the other side.

Continue switching sides for twenty to thirty seconds, rest for ten seconds, then repeat two to three more rounds if you like.

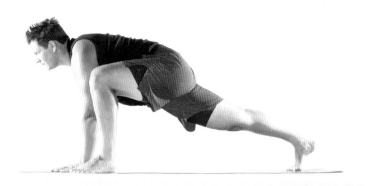

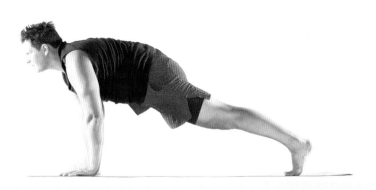

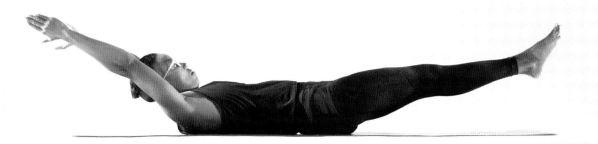

Hollow Hold

Purpose: To develop core strength and stability. (This is particularly useful for those of us with the common tendency to overarch our lower backs in handstand, which can make it difficult to hold!)

In Practice: Lie on your back, curl your head and shoulders up off the mat, keeping a little bit of space between your chin and your chest, and hold on to the back of your right thigh with your right hand. Stretch your left leg out long, high enough from the floor that you don't arch your lower back significantly. Hold for fifteen to thirty seconds before switching sides.

To intensify, you can stretch both legs long at once (as Shanté is in the photo), either keeping your arms alongside you or reaching them up alongside your ears to intensify further. Hold this variation for thirty to sixty seconds.

Tip: If this pose bothers your neck, place one hand behind your head. And it might sound weird but pressing your tongue into the roof of your mouth can also help to take pressure out of your neck!

Pigeon Variation

Purpose: To increase hip flexibility.

In Practice: From downward-facing dog or hands and knees, bring your left shin forward so your left knee is near your left wrist and your left ankle is near your right wrist. Point your front foot but flex the toes back toward you so that your foot is in between flexed and pointed, and press the pinky-toe side of your foot into the floor so that your front ankle is straight (not collapsing inward).

Draw your left hip back and right hip forward until you start to feel a stretch. Stretch your right leg behind you so that you're resting on the bottom of the thigh in the front kneecap. You can point your back foot or tuck your back toes under. You can remain upright or fold forward, perhaps bringing your forearms to the floor in front of you or stretching your arms straight ahead.

Stay for one minute, then bring your torso upright if you were in the fold and slide your front leg back to return to your starting position. Then switch sides.

Firelog Pose (*Agnistambhasana*)

Purpose: To increase hip flexibility. You may find you prefer this stretch to pigeon, or vice versa! Try experimenting with both in your practice.

In Practice: Sit tall on the floor. If your lower back rounds, sit on the edge of a folded blanket or two in order to establish a neutral spine where your lower back curves in slightly.

Bend your left knee and, with your left foot flexed, move your left shin so that it's roughly parallel to the top edge of your mat (bent at about a ninety-degree angle). Then bend your right knee and stack your right shin on top of your left, right foot flexed too, so your right ankle is on top of your left knee and your right foot is off your thigh.

Either remain upright or fold forward.

Stay for a few breaths, or longer if you'd like, then rise up if you were folding forward and switch sides.

Tips: If your top knee is higher than you'd like and it's uncomfortable, you can place a prop under it, such as a bolster or a folded blanket. Another option is to place a block in front of your bottom shin and rest your top foot or ankle on the block.

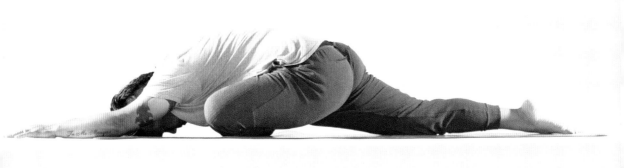
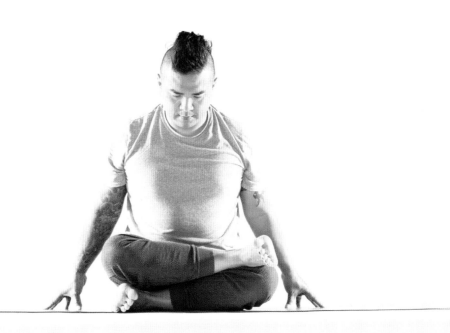

Seated Wide-Legged Forward Fold

Purpose: To stretch your hips, inner thighs, and hamstrings.

In Practice: Sit tall on your mat with your legs out in front of you, feet flexed. If your lower back rounds, sit up on a folded blanket or two to find a neutral spine. Separate your legs wide—wide enough that you'll feel a stretch through your inner thighs when you start to hinge forward, but not so wide that you can't keep your knees and toes pointing up toward the ceiling.

Inhale, lengthen your spine. Exhale, hinge at your hips and start to walk your hands forward between your legs. Keep your spine long and stop where you start to feel a good stretch, knees and toes still pointing up. At some point your spine might round, and if you get to that point, let your lower and middle back round too, and aim to find a little bit more length through your upper back. (Often the upper back tends to round a lot more in forward folds.) Stay for five to ten breaths, and on an inhale, return upright.

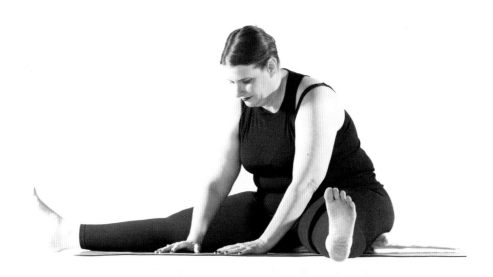

Garland Pose (*Malasana*), a.k.a. "a Squat"

Purpose: To stretch your hips, ankles, and calves.

In Practice: Come into a squat with your feet a comfortable distance apart (this varies greatly from person to person) and your knees and toes pointing in the same direction. If it's comfortable, let your hips sink low, below the level of your knees. If it's not, keep your hips at or above knee level. If your heels don't reach the floor, support them with a rolled mat or blanket, like Kyle.

Bring your hands to your heart, and perhaps your elbows inside your knees. You can use your elbows to press your knees outward, keeping your knees pointing in the same direction as your toes. Lengthen through your torso and stay here for five to ten breaths.

To come out, place your hands on the ground or a prop, lift your hips if you lowered them below your knees, and come into a standing forward bend. Stay there for a few breaths, then rise to standing.

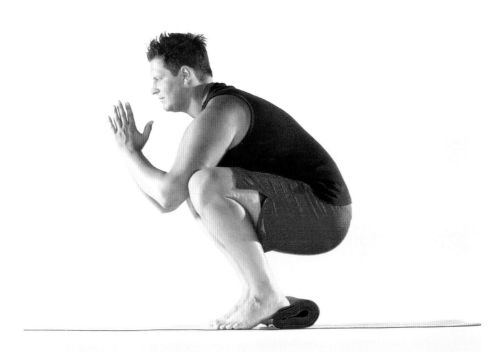

Handstand (Adho Mukha Vrksasana)

Walking Up into Handstand at the Wall

This step-by-step approach (which I first learned from my fellow yoga teacher and friend Allison Jeraci) will help you take your downward-facing dog into a handstand by gradually transferring more weight into your hands and helping you to get your hips up over your shoulders. Shifting weight into the hands and getting the hips up high are common challenges that many of us face when learning how to handstand. The key here is to (quite literally) take it one step at a time and gradually increase the load you're asking your upper body to bear and the amount of height under your feet over time.

————

Set up the short edge of your mat against the wall and have two to four yoga blocks on hand. Set up two blocks on their shortest height, about your own hips-width apart (or as wide as you like your feet to be in downward-facing dog), with the short edges touching the wall.

I recommend starting with two blocks, and then if you feel comfortable there and you'd like to get a feel for getting your hips up higher—closer to where they would be in a handstand—you can stack two more blocks on top of those. (Note that in the photo below, Shanté is using "double thick" blocks that are the same height as two stacked sets of blocks.)

Once set up, come into downward-facing dog with the balls of your feet on the blocks and your heels touching the wall. Stay here for several breaths.

Notice how the added height under your feet shifts more weight into your hands.

Tip: If one of your main hand-balancing goals is to increase your upper-body strength/ability to weight-bear, try holding this or any of these at-the-wall handstand variations for time. Perhaps start with ten seconds and work your way up to a minute. If a minute starts to feel "easy" in the block variation, try the chair variation next; then if a minute with the chair starts to feel "easy," try holding the L-pose variation for time (see page 44).

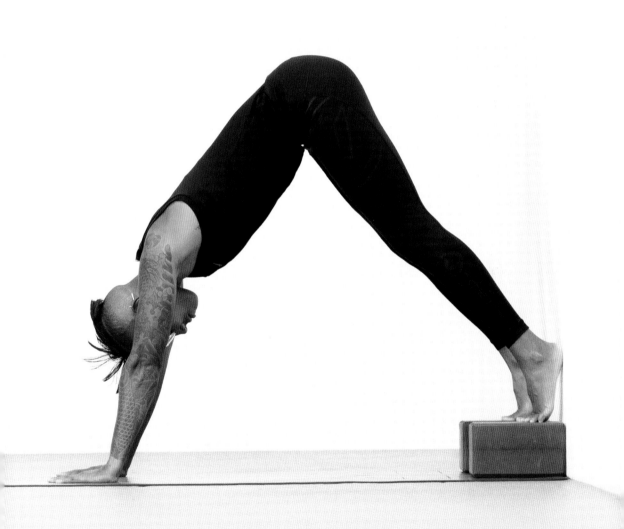

Chair Variation

If you'd like to begin transferring more weight into your upper body and lifting your hips up higher—more over your shoulders—moving even closer toward a vertical handstand, try this variation with a chair (another great variation I picked up from Allison when we were working together at Yoga International):

———

With your mat at the wall, set up a sturdy chair about the distance of one of your leg's length away from the wall, or perhaps just a bit farther away (see the following L-pose variation to see how to measure this in more detail), with the seat facing toward the wall.

Facing the wall, plant your hands on the mat so that your fingertips are about a palm's distance away from the wall and walk the balls of your feet onto the chair seat. (Finding your ideal distance and the chair's ideal distance from the wall may take some trial and error, so come out of the pose and adjust as needed.) Remain here for several breaths and notice what it feels like to have your hips up a lot higher—almost right over your shoulders—and even more weight in your hands while still in a supported position.

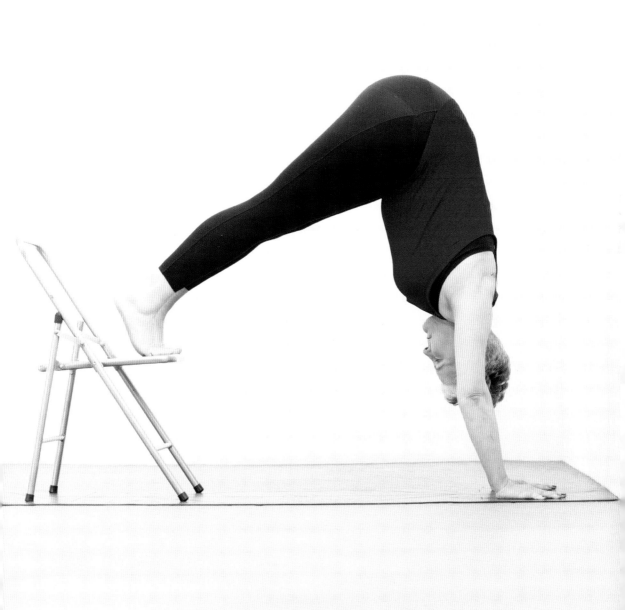

L Pose at the Wall

Ready to bring even more weight into your hands and get your hips *right* up over your shoulders? Then it's time to explore L pose at the wall. This variation actually requires *more* weight-bearing through your upper body than a middle-of-the-room handstand, so you'll be extra prepared on that front! But because you're still "walking" up into it and your feet are pressing into the wall, you have more control over the transition than you would hopping or jumping into handstand, making this variation a little less scary for a lot of folks.

———

To set up, sit with your back against the wall and your legs straight out in front of you, feet flexed, as Nam is demonstrating in the photo. Notice where your heels are, and place a marker, such as a block or strap, there. This is your "legs' length" distance from the wall.

Once you've measured your legs' length, come to hands and knees, facing away from the wall, with the heels of your hands right about where your heels were when you measured (move your marker out of the way if needed). Tuck your toes, lift your knees, and begin to walk your feet up the wall, stopping when your heels get to hip height. Ideally you want your shoulders right over your wrists here. As with the previous variation, you may need to come down and adjust your distance from the wall a bit until you find your own ideal placement from which to begin. Once you've found your optimal distance from the wall—where you can walk up into the pose with your heels right about at hip height, your hips over your shoulders, and your shoulders over your wrists—stay here for a few breaths. Push your heels into the wall and push your hands into the floor, as though you were "pushing the ground away." These actions can help you find more stability and ease in the pose, keep your feet from slipping, and prevent you from "dumping" your bodyweight into your shoulders (which is not super comfortable).

Walk your feet back down the wall when you're ready to come out.

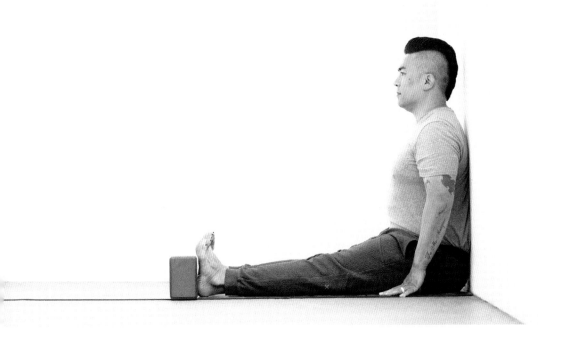

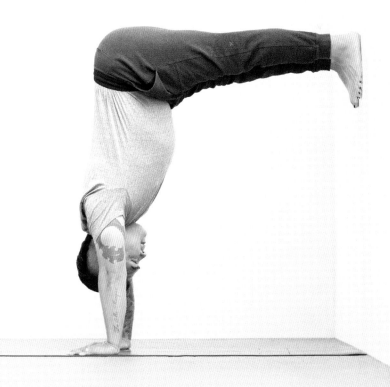

Hopping Into Handstand

If you're just learning to hop into handstand or if you're concerned about flipping over, I suggest practicing at the wall, with the short edge of your mat right up against it as in the previous variations. Try setting up with your fingertips about a palm print away from the wall. As you get more comfortable with your balance, you can move farther from the wall.

"Hoption" 1: One Knee Bent

Set up in a short downward-facing dog (facing the wall if you're using one).

Step your left foot forward, toward the top of your mat, so there's about one foot of space between your foot and your hands.

Lift your back leg up and rise onto the ball of your right foot, shifting your shoulders forward so that they're stacked over your wrists or even slightly forward of your wrists. (Depending on your proportions, you may need to scoot your bottom foot forward a bit more to do this.) Gaze toward your hands.

Note: You don't have to keep your hips square for this variation. If it feels good, let your lifted (right) leg turn out a little. (Some folks find that this makes the hopping easier!)

This is your setup for the handstand hop, but before you "hop to it," try this prep to get comfortable with the movements:

Inhale to prepare.

Exhale, bend your left knee and tap your right toes on the floor, keeping your gaze toward your hands.

Inhale, straighten your left leg and float your right leg back up.

Repeat this a few times. Then, if you like, you can add in the hop:

Inhale, lift your right leg.

Exhale, bend your left knee and tap your right toes to the mat.

Then, briefly suspend your exhale and hop up, bending your left knee in toward your chest.

Repeat this a few more times. Eventually you might catch a little "hang time" in a handstand! If you're practicing at a wall, you can bring one or both heels to the wall. Lower one leg at time to come down.

Then switch sides and try a few rounds hopping off of your right foot.

Variation: If suspending your exhale for the hop feels awkward, try this breathing pattern instead: inhale, lift your back leg; exhale, tap and hop.

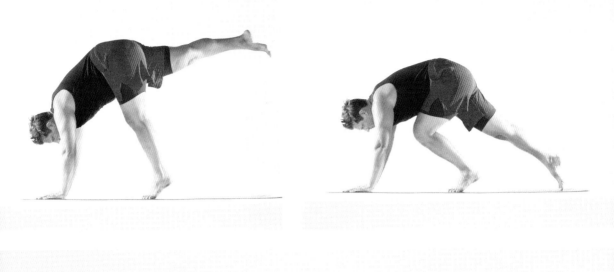

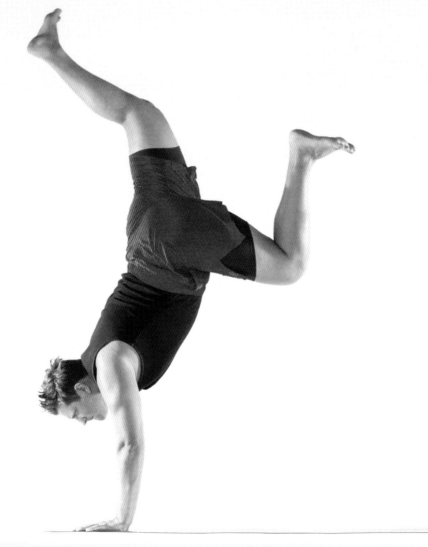

"Hoption" 2: Both Legs Straight (L-Shape Variation)

Set up the same way as "hoption" 1, in a short downward-facing dog.

Step your right foot forward (we'll start by hopping off the opposite foot this time) so there's about a foot of space between your foot and hands. Lift your left leg and rise onto the ball of your right foot, shifting your shoulders over or slightly past your wrists. Gaze toward your hands. This is your starting position for the hops.

Unlike "hoption" 1, you'll keep your hips relatively square to the ground; and instead of tapping your back toes to the floor, you'll keep your left leg lifted.

Inhale to prepare.

Exhale, bend your right knee and hop up. Lead with your hips to come into an L-shape handstand. Repeat a few times. If you happen to catch some hang time, you can bring your right leg to meet your left for a vertical handstand. Lower one leg at a time to come down.

Then switch sides and try a few rounds hopping off of your left foot.

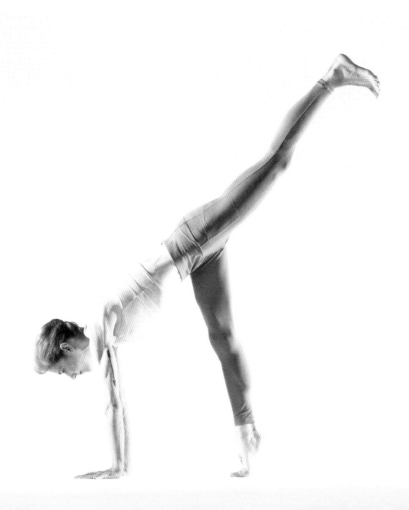

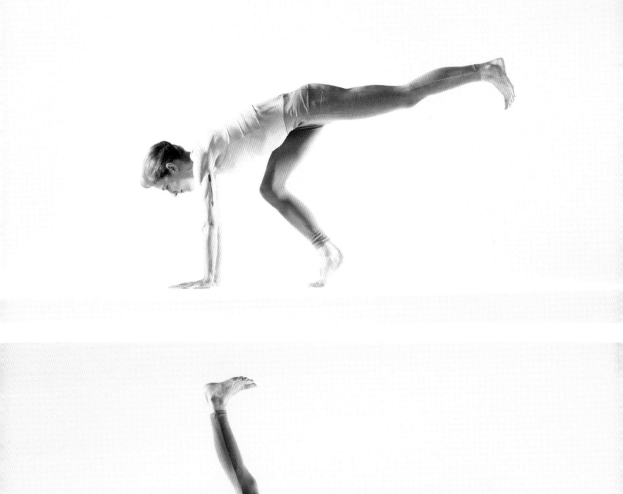
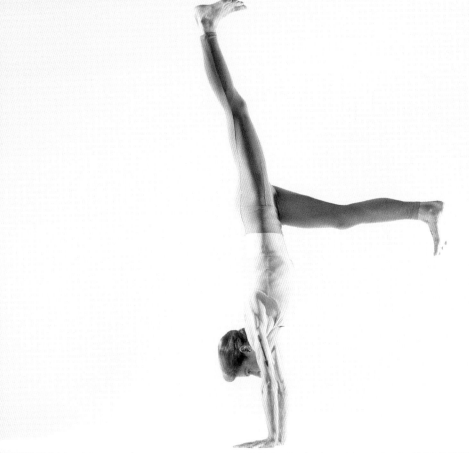

Jumping Into Handstand

So what's the difference between a hop and a jump? I'm glad you asked! Though sometimes the terms are used interchangeably, you "hop" off of one foot and land on one foot, and you "jump" off of both feet and land on both feet.

Some folks find hopping more accessible, while others prefer jumping. One of the added perks of jumping is that it's a great skill-builder for "floating forward" to the top of your mat in a sun salutation or other vinyasa transition (page 88).

———

Set up in—you guessed it—a short downward-facing dog. I like to step my feet together to jump into handstand, but other people prefer feet apart. Try both and see what works for you.

On an inhale, rise onto the balls of your feet and gaze toward your hands.

Exhale, bend your knees and jump up, kicking your heels to your seat (aim to get your hips up over your shoulders). Land in a bent-knee downward-facing dog and repeat these "tuck jumps" (also sometimes called "cannonballs" or "donkey kicks") several times.

Tip: If you're practicing at a wall, it can be helpful to aim your hips toward the wall.

If (like Nam in the photo) you're able to catch hang time in your handstand, you can bring your legs into a butterfly position—a nice shape for securing your balance before you straighten your legs.

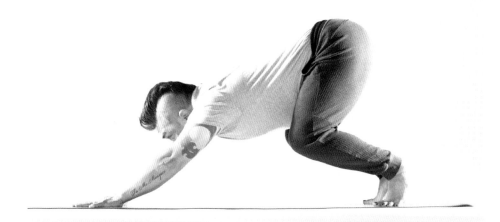

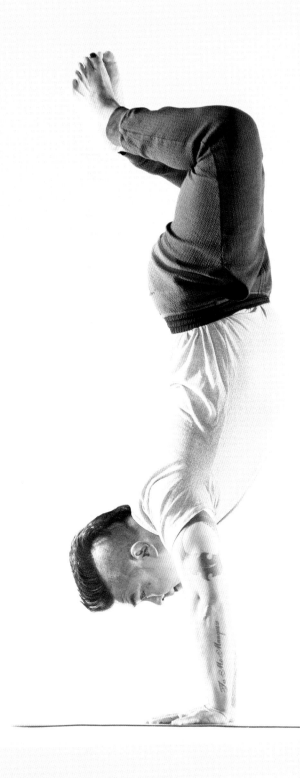

Alternative: "The Gymnastics Way" with a Bolster at the Wall

As someone who learned to handstand in yoga class, with downward-facing dog as the foundation, coming into a handstand from standing—planting my hands and kicking right up—seemed pretty terrifying to me initially. This is why I was surprised when a friend of mine, who had struggled with the "yoga approach" to handstands for a long time, shared that she was finally able to handstand confidently after learning to come into it in what she called "the gymnastics way" with a bolster at the wall. She showed me this approach, which another teacher had shown her, and since then I've offered it as an alternative for students who don't particularly enjoy coming into handstand from downward-facing dog.

And no matter how you come into it, working with a bolster at the wall in this way can be helpful for getting a sense of what it feels like to handstand with both feet off the wall while still being in a supported position.

———

To set up, you'll once again place the short edge of your mat against a wall. Place a bolster right up against the wall, vertically (a stiffer bolster will work best for this variation).

Before you kick up into handstand, note where you'll place your hands. The exact position will depend on the thickness of your bolster, but in general, you want to make sure that when you kick up, the back of your head comes in contact with the bolster and your heels can (initially) touch the wall. A good starting place might be to plant your hands just a little bit in front of the end of the bolster farthest from the wall, as Shanté is doing in the photo.

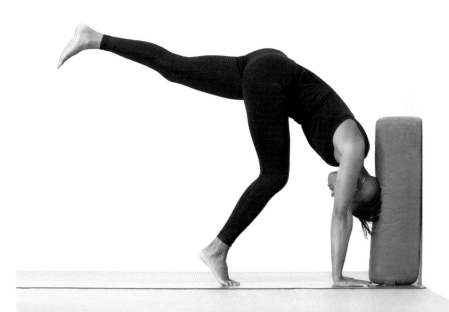

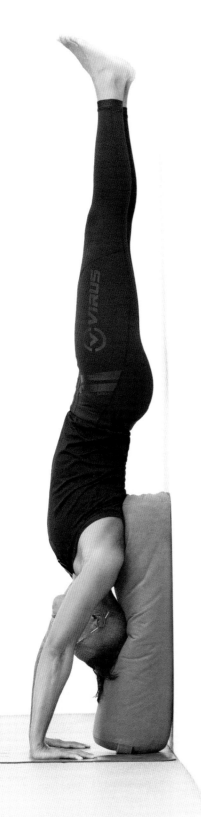

Once you've found that starting place for your hands, stand back behind the bolster, far enough away that you can plant your hands and kick up. Reach your arms up overhead with your palms facing the wall. Point your right foot forward, as you would if you were going to do a cartwheel. Inhale to prepare, and as you exhale, step with your right foot, plant your hands, and kick up, bringing your heels to the wall.

Once you're there, flex your feet. Press the back of your head into the bolster and press your hands into the floor, like you're pushing the ground away from you. At the same time, reach your inner heels up toward the ceiling and see if you can float them off of the wall. The back of your head pressing into the bolster and the actions of pressing your hands into the ground while reaching up through your inner heels will help you stay supported in the pose.

Stay for a few breaths if possible, then lower one leg at a time to come down.

HOW TO TAKE YOUR HANDSTAND OFF THE WALL (IF YOU WANT TO)

Here are some tips to get you started!

- Start by moving your mat away from the wall a little bit at a time—far enough away that you don't immediately touch it with your heels when you hop up but close enough that you'll still touch it easily if you lose your balance. Over time, as you grow more confident in your ability to balance, you can move it even farther.

- Don't bring your legs together right away. If you hop up into handstand, keep your legs apart as you find your balance, and only join your legs together once you feel stable.

- In general, if you feel like you're going to flip over into a backbend, try shifting more weight into your fingertips.

- Also in general, if you feel like you're going to fall back toward a downward-facing dog, try shifting more weight into the heels of your hands.

- Spread your toes! This tiny little "activation" can make a big difference.

SAMPLE ONE-MONTH PLAN FOR TAKING YOUR HANDSTAND OFF THE WALL

- Choose any three days each week to do these practices every week for one month.

- Feel free to swap out drills and stretches as needed to best align with your needs and goals!

See "Taking Your Handstand Off the Wall" tables in appendix 1 starting on page 176.

PRESSING UP INTO HANDSTAND

The "quest for the press" is a goal for a lot of yoga practitioners. Why? Well, for one, it does look pretty impressive to "effortlessly" float into a handstand from a standing forward fold without using any momentum. But from a practical point of view, it's a less haphazard, more controlled way to approach a handstand. Because momentum isn't involved as it is when hopping or jumping up, it's easier to put on the brakes and come into the inversion slowly. So even though for most of us it's a more difficult transition to learn, once you learn it (at least in my experience) it's a less "scary" way to enter your handstands.

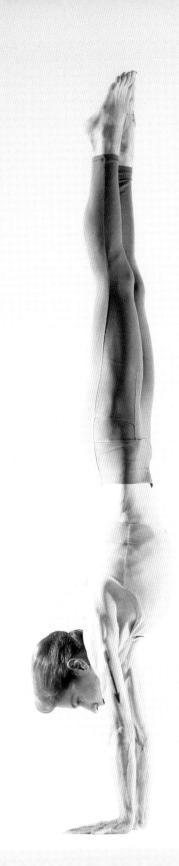

And the benefits don't stop there! Because it requires a heck of a lot of upper-body and core strength, handstand press and the skills and drills you practice to get there are fabulous upper-body and core-strengthening exercises! Let's explore a few standouts:

Toe/Heel Rocks

Some key factors that help a *lot* when it comes to pressing up include shifting weight into your fingertips and pressing your hands strongly into the ground (this helps you get your hips up over your shoulders and your tippy-toes off the floor) and having open hamstrings (this will definitely put you at an advantage and give you a little extra "oomph" for getting your hips over your shoulders). This drill will help with both.

Begin in a standing forward bend with your hands either planted on the floor or on blocks. (If using blocks, grip them with your fingers and thumbs on all sides and think of them as extensions of your arms. It's okay for the blocks to move as you do, just as your hands might if they were flat on the floor.)

Start with your hands or blocks about a foot or less in front of your feet. Though it might feel tempting to have them way more forward, closer in like this will make it

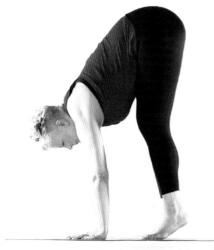
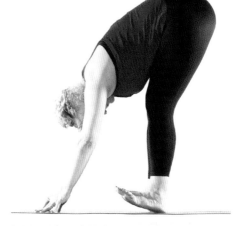

easier to transfer weight into your fingertips and (eventually) get your hips up over your shoulders. It's fine to bend your knees for this drill.

Gaze forward toward your hands and, on an inhale, rock up onto your tippy-toes as high as you possibly can.

On an exhale, rock back onto your heels to stretch your hamstrings. You can walk your hands/blocks forward if you like, perhaps coming up onto your fingertips, and you can allow your back to round, relaxing your head and neck, if that feels good.

Repeat this drill a few times: inhale, planting your hands firmly and rocking forward onto your tiptoes; exhale, rocking back onto your heels.

––––––––

Once that starts to feel easy, you can add in the toe-taps. This helps to bring even more weight into your upper body and brings you even closer to a handstand press!

As with the previous variation, inhale, rock forward onto your tiptoes as high as you can. On your exhale, try to pick up your right foot and tap your right toes to—or as close as you can get to—your right wrist (or block).

Inhale, return your right foot to its starting place.

Exhale, tap your left toes to or toward your left wrist (or block).

Inhale, return your left foot to its starting place.

Exhale, rock back onto your heels, stretching your hamstrings and releasing your back.

Repeat a few more rounds like this.

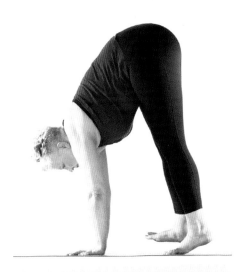 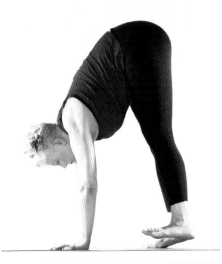

Press Walks

Press walks are a popular handstand drill for a reason. They're effective! These, too, provide a great hamstring stretch and help you get accustomed to shifting weight into your fingertips and pressing your hands into the ground.

———

Begin near the top of your mat, with your hands planted about a foot or less in front of your feet. (Bend your knees as much as you need to in order to plant your hands.)

Gaze forward toward your hands.

On an inhale, rise up onto your tiptoes, shifting weight into your fingertips and "pressing the ground away."

Exhale, step one foot back and then the other.

Then walk your hands back so that they're once again a foot or less in front of your feet. Repeat the press walk until you reach the back of your mat.

You can conclude the drill here, walk to the front of your mat and repeat it, or try "press walking" forward to the top of your mat. (You may want to start with your hands a little more forward for the forward walks. Experiment with their placement and see what works for you.)

Over time, your "walks" might turn more into "floats," and you may even be able to hover both feet off the floor at some point!

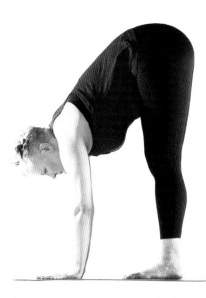

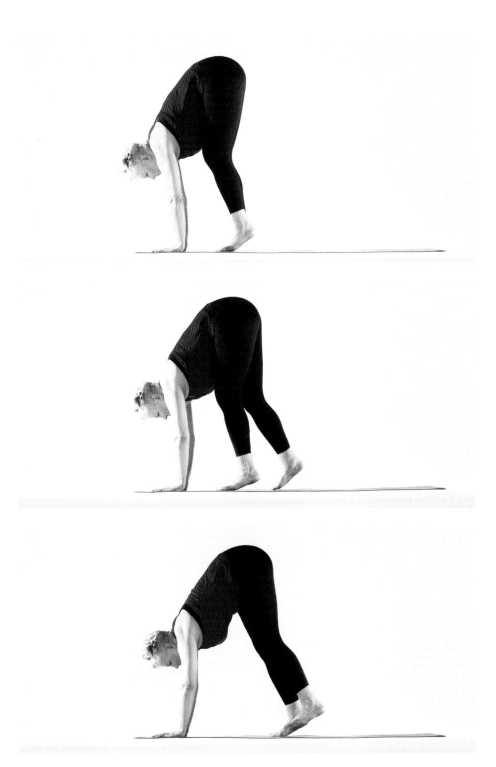

Toe-Tap Drill with Chair

I discovered this drill after I learned to handstand press, and my first thought was "Where have you been all my life?" I'm pretty sure I would have "completed" that "quest for the press" a lot sooner had I been practicing this regularly! The chair helps you get your hips up super high and transfer more weight into your hands.

———

Place all four legs of a sturdy chair onto a mat to prevent it from slipping. Turn the seat to face you and then come onto your mat with your back facing the chair. Plant your hands on the mat and step your feet up onto the chair, one at a time, to come into a downward-facing-dog-type setup, as Nam is demonstrating in the photo.

Adjust your positioning as needed so that your wrists are right under your shoulders. (This is key!) Rise up onto the balls of your feet and walk them as close to the edge of the chair as you can. Gaze toward your hands.

Inhale, lift your left leg in the air.

Exhale, try to tap your left toes to or toward your left wrist. (You can bend your right knee as you do this, but keep your left leg straight.)

Inhale, reach your left leg back up, and straighten your right leg again.

Try a couple more taps on the left side. Take a break if you need to, then repeat on the right.

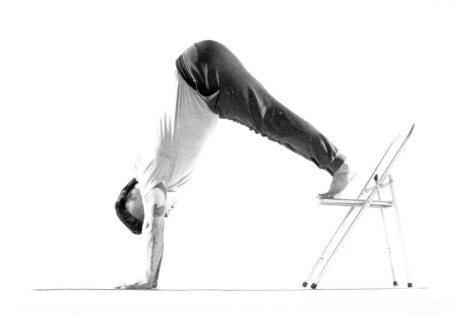

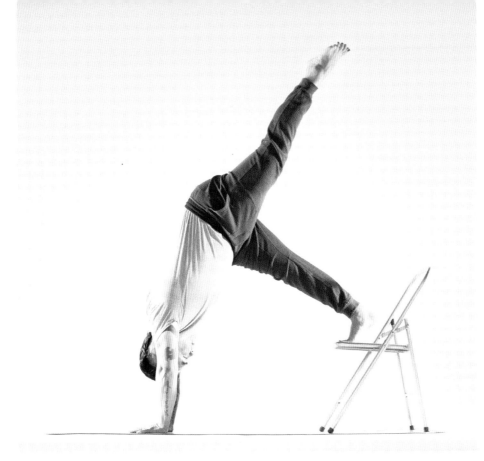

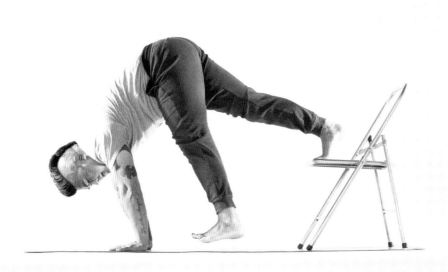

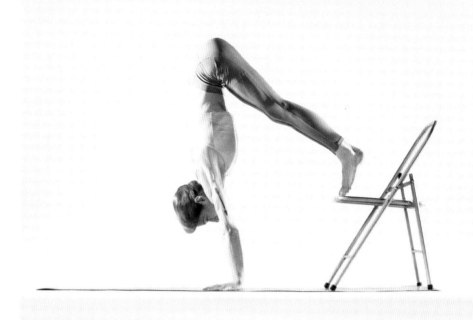

Straddle Press

So you've done your drills and you feel ready to try a press! Where to begin?

———

I recommend starting with a straddle press (pressing up with your legs wide apart), with a whole lot of height underneath your feet to start. The chair version pictured above and described below is a great option.

It's also a great press variation in general if your hips and hamstrings are on the tighter side or if you have long limbs and a short torso, which naturally tends to make pressing more challenging because it requires you to recruit more shoulder strength and hamstring flexibility than your long-torsoed, short-limbed friends. The chair quite literally levels the playing field!

With a Chair

Note: Before you attempt this one in the middle of the room as pictured, make sure you're super confident in your handstands in general and that you're comfortable "cartwheeling" your legs off to the side to fall out. You can also work with an experienced spotter. If middle of the room isn't in the cards yet, but you're still ready and raring to press, practice with your back facing a wall.

———

Begin as you did for the toe-tap drill with a chair, in a downward-facing-dog-like position, with your shoulders over your wrists, your feet on the chair (close to the edge), and your gaze toward your hands. Rise up *super* high on your toes to really get your hips up over your shoulders.

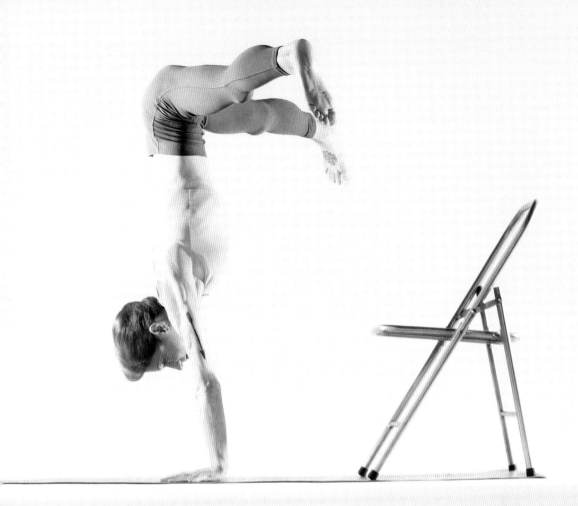

Breathe in whatever way feels most comfortable and natural to you. (I like to lift up high on my toes on the inhale and to try to press up on the exhale.)

As you rise high onto your toes, shift more weight into your fingertips and get your hips up even higher!

As your toes get lighter and lighter, you might be able to float them off of the chair, separating your legs wide, in a straddle. (This position can give you that little extra leverage to get your hips up and can initially be easier to balance in.)

You can try lifting just one leg at first, perhaps opening just your right leg out to the side (press into your left hand to stay balanced). From there you can lower your right foot back down and repeat on your left side, or, if it feels right, float your left leg up and out to the side to match your right.

Or if you're feeling it, you can lift and straddle both legs together as I am in the photo above.

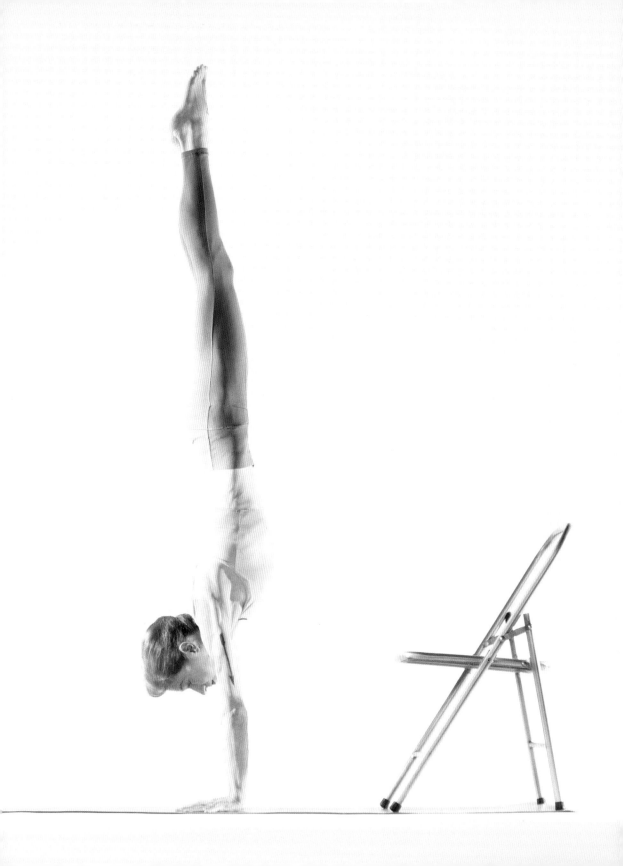

If you feel really stable, you can join your legs together in the air.

Come down before you feel like you "have to," either lowering one foot at a time to the chair or straddling your legs again (if they were together) and slowly, with control, lowering both feet to the ground behind your hands.

With Blocks

If the chair feels "easy," try your straddle press with less height under your feet—perhaps using blocks, as Nam is in the following photo.

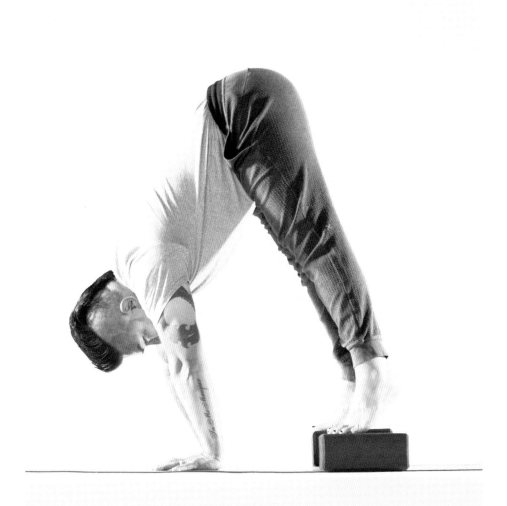

Without Props

If pressing off of blocks begins to feel "easy," try a straddle press sans props. To set yourself up for success, start with your hands close to your feet (about a foot or less in front of them) and gaze toward your hands.

Some people like to begin their straddle press with their legs really close together and then widen their legs out to the side as they come up. Others like to start with their feet a little wider—say, hip-width apart—and still others prefer to start with their legs *really* wide in a wide-legged forward bend.

Experiment with different entrances and see what feels best in your body. (This may change on the daily!)

Rise up high onto your tiptoes, shifting more and more and *more* weight into your fingertips as you push the ground away from you.

Aim to get your hips *up* over your shoulders as you get *really* light on your toes, maybe even floating them off the ground as you straddle your legs wide and press up.

If you feel stable, bring your legs together, and when you're ready to come down, straddle your legs again and aim to lower both feet to the floor with as much control as you used to press up!

Tip: If you aren't yet able to press up but are comfortable coming into a handstand another way, "pressing down" (also known as "working the negative") by straddling your legs and lowering both feet to floor together slowly and with control is a really effective way to develop your pressing skills.

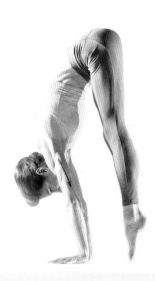

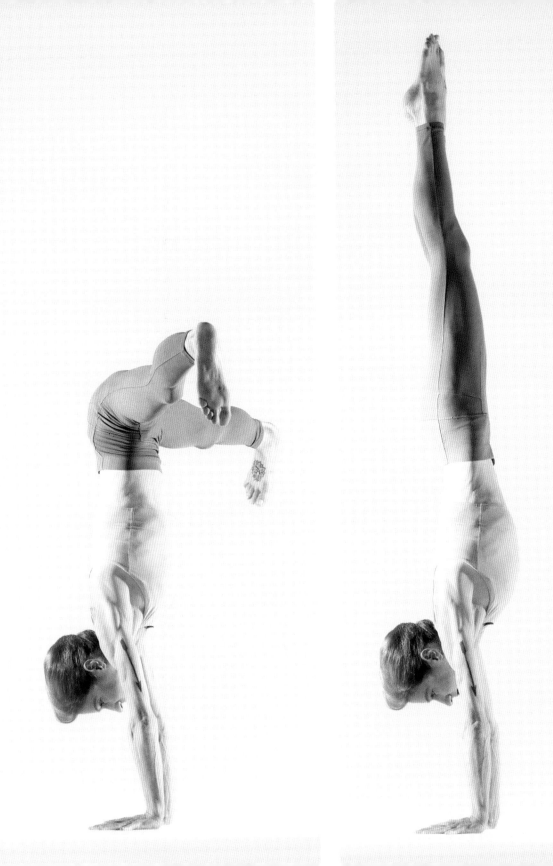

Toe-Tap Hover Drills to Finesse Your Press

These drills are great for continuing to hone your pressing skills as you work toward more challenging variations like pike presses, and if you're still working toward a straddle press, they are pretty effective there too—especially when it comes to building the necessary upper-body strength. These babies are *killer* (in a good way)!

You can think of this as a progression of the heel rock/toe-tap drill with the toe-taps we explored beginning on page 56.

Begin just as you did for the straddle press: in a forward bend with your hands planted fairly close to your feet. For this one, though, start with your feet no wider than your hands.

Gaze forward toward your hands, and on an inhale, rise up high onto your toes.

Exhale, tap your left toes to or toward your left wrist or forearm, as high up as you can.

You can return your left foot to its starting position and repeat on the other side, or keep your left foot there and see if you can float your right toes up too (*keep* shifting weight into your fingertips!) and bring your right toes to your right wrist or forearm.

Lower your feet to the floor and repeat, perhaps starting with the right foot next.

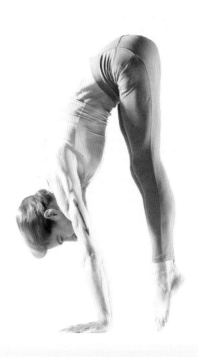

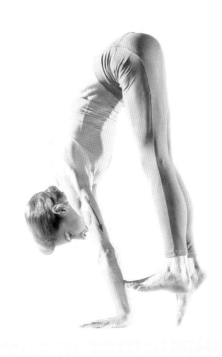

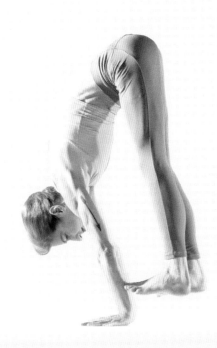

Variation 1: If your hamstrings feel tight and/or the previous variation doesn't quite work for your proportions, practicing with your feet on blocks and your knees bent may be helpful.

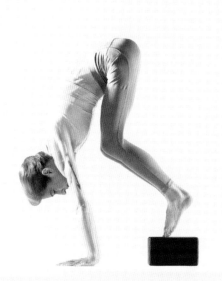
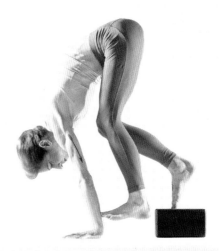
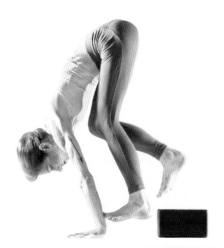
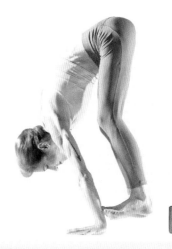

Variation 2: Instead of tapping one foot at a time, you can also try bringing both feet to your wrists/forearms simultaneously, either without blocks and/or bent knees or with them.

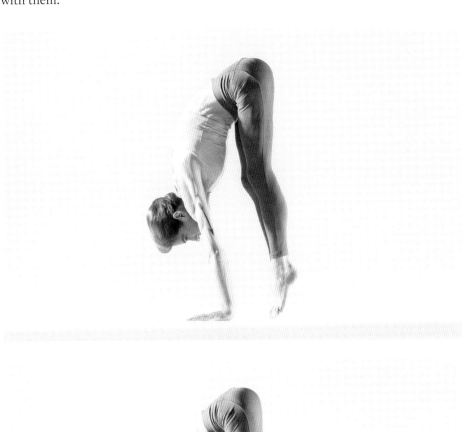

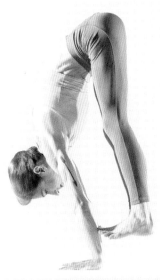

Toe-Tap Press

To progress your toe-to-wrist taps further, take it to a handstand press. (If your feet are already off the ground/blocks, why not?)

———

With your toes at your forearms/wrists, continue shifting your weight forward, pushing the ground away, and straddle your legs wide to come up.

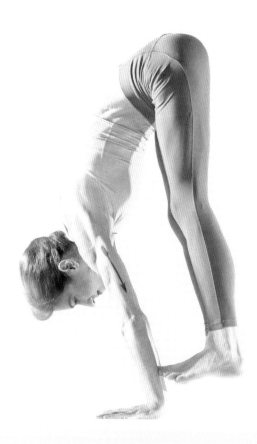

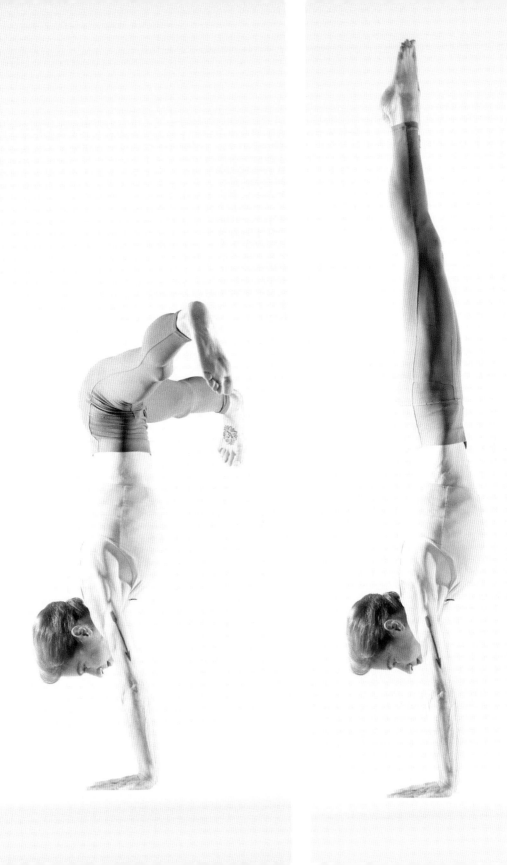

If you're keeping your knees bent (as I am in the following photos), they can stay bent as you straddle.

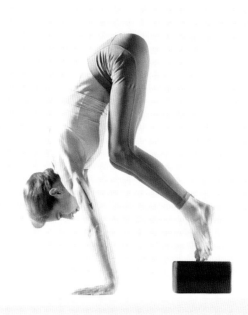

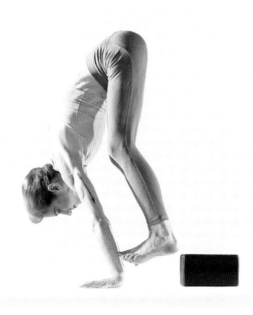

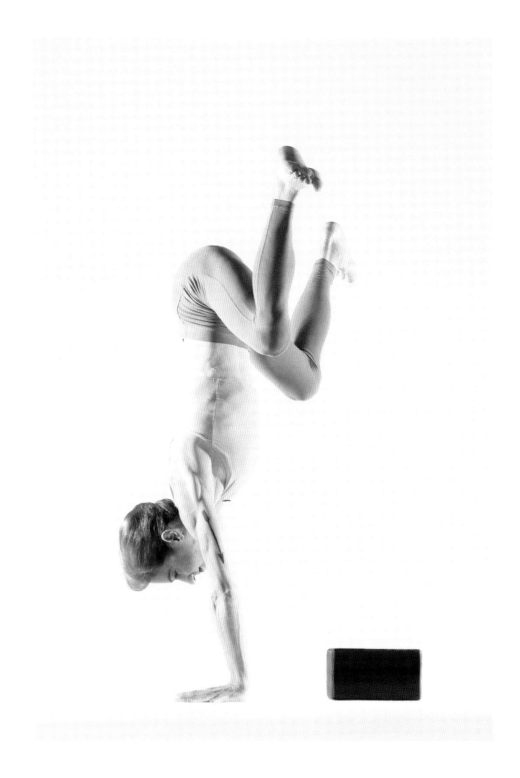

One-Footed Press Variations

The more I practice and teach yoga, the more I realize that every body is wonderfully unique! For me, the straddle is usually "easiest," probably due to the fact that I have a long torso, short limbs, and pretty flexible hips and hamstrings. (Don't ask me about my backbends, though, please! Those do not come so easily for my proportions . . . but you can check out my previous book, *Yoga Where You Are*, cowritten with Dianne Bondy, to see how I learned to [sort of] like them.)

For many of my handstanding friends, though—with different bodies, different proportions, and different strengths and challenges—one-footed press variations tend to come easier.

Puppy Press

The puppy press in particular is often a great variation to start with: one leg is already in the air, and the external rotation of the hip joint, combined with the bent knee, can provide additional leverage that makes it easier to float the bottom foot up.

As with the straddle press, you can get some extra lift from a chair or a block (as Nam is demonstrating in the photos).

(And yes, it *is* called a puppy press because you take a similar shape to the one many dogs take to . . . relieve themselves. Embrace it. No one ever said handstands had to be serious.)

———

Here, too, start with your hands planted about a foot or so in front of your feet. Lift your left leg in the air and come onto the ball of your right foot as you shift your shoulders over your wrists, gazing toward your hands.

Let your left hip open up, lifting your leg as much as feels good, and bend your knee (like you might to "flip your dog" into wild thing pose in a yoga class).

Continue to shift more weight into your fingertips and push the ground away—maybe your right toes float up!

If they do, extend your right leg out to the side in a straddle position and then straighten your left leg, extending it out to the side so that you're in a full straddle.

Stay there, or if you feel stable, draw your legs together if you'd like.

Lower one foot at a time to come out. If you're using a chair or a block, aim to land your right foot first, exactly where it started on the prop.

Be sure to try the other side too. You will likely find that one side is a little easier than the other.

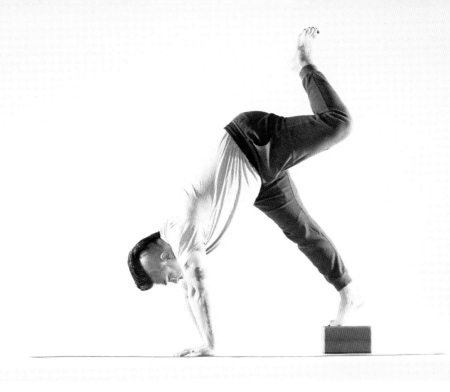

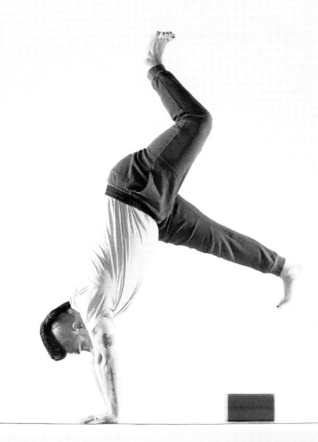

Tip: If the press isn't happening just yet, try hopping your bottom foot up (just a *little* hop) and as you do, still push the floor away and shift your weight forward, which will help you get your hips up over your shoulders and prepare you for the puppy press. Over time, you might find that your hop magically turns into a press.

Single Straight-Leg Press

You can also try a single-foot press with both legs straight (or close to straight). As with the puppy press, feel free to elevate your bottom foot with a prop if you like.

As in previous variations, plant your hands, gaze toward them, and shift a ton of weight into your fingertips. Aim to shift your shoulders *past* your wrists, and as you push the ground away, try to float your toes off the floor or your prop.

You can open the hip of your top leg as much as feels good for you. Be sure to do both sides.

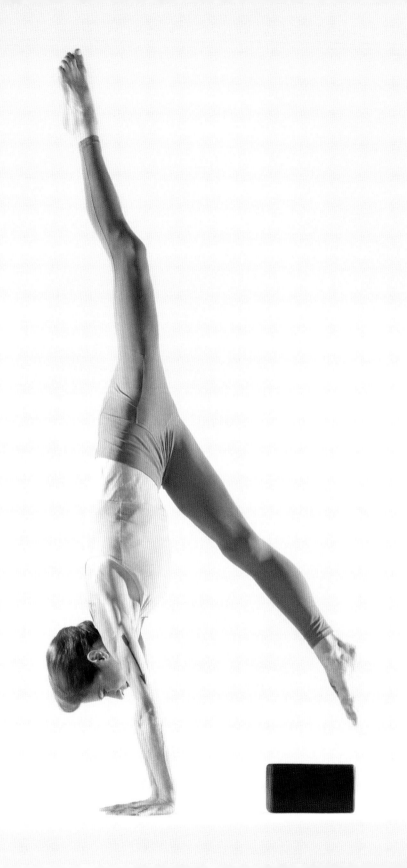

Single-Leg Tuck Press

If you're working toward a pike press (page 83), this one-footed tuck-press variation is a great prep and skill-builder. (It's also a pretty cool variation in its own right!)

———

Set up as you did the previous single-leg press variations, incorporating any props that you'd like. As you rise up onto your right (your pressing leg) toes and shift your shoulders forward, gazing forward, bend your left heel in toward your seat.

When your right toes float up, draw your right heel in toward your seat as well, coming into a full tuck position.

If you find your balance in the tuck, feel free to straighten your legs for a "traditional" handstand shape, or explore any other leg variation you like! Release as you like and try the other side.

Progression: If you're using this as a pike-press prep, once the previous variation feels comfortable, try keeping your right leg (your pressing leg) straight the whole way up. (In a pike press, you'll do this with both legs straight.) Then switch sides.

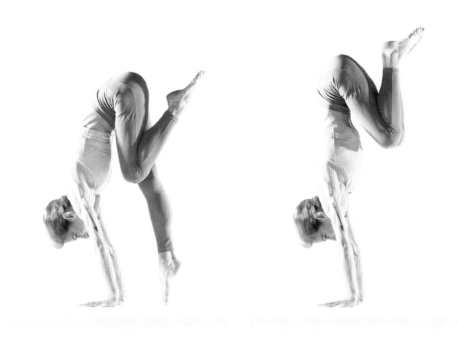

Two-Footed Press Variations

Every body is different, but speaking in general, the variations that follow are ones that folks typically explore after working with a straddle press (page 62) and/or the single-leg press variations we looked at previously. That's because they typically require more "raw" upper-body strength, as you don't get as much help from your hip and hamstring flexibility in getting your hips up over your shoulders.

That said, if you have a lot of upper-body strength (especially when it comes to "pushing" exercises like handstands) and less hip and hamstring flexibility, you may find that they come easier for you! Particularly the two-footed tuck press that follows.

———

Set up as you did in the previous press variations, with or without a prop under your feet. For this one, you'll want your feet pretty close together (as close as they comfortably can be, generally speaking).

Shift lots of weight into your fingertips and push the floor away, coming as high up onto your toes as you can until (maybe!) your toes float off the floor or prop.

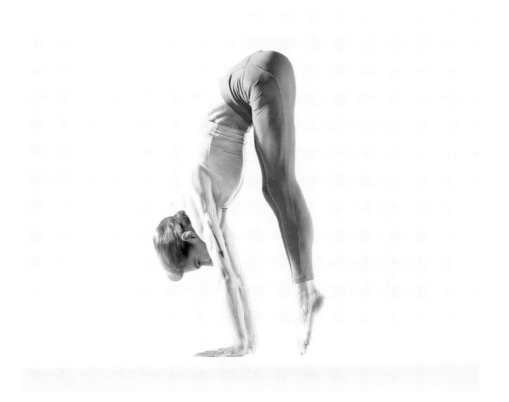

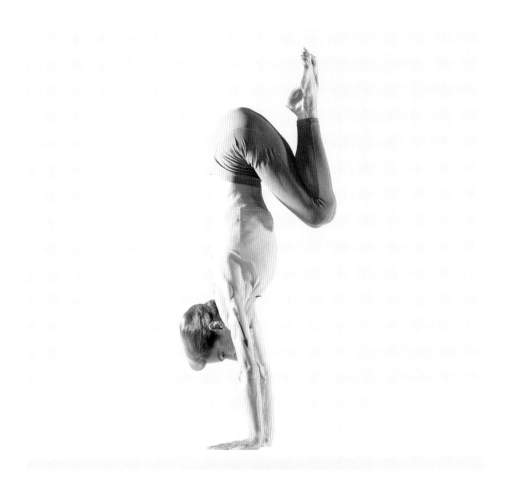

Then bend both knees together. (This can help you get your hips even *more* up over your shoulders, perhaps giving you just the boost you need to really "stick" the handstand!) Stay here or, if you find your balance, explore any leg variation you like before coming down.

Tip: If you're working toward a pike press, you can build strength and skills by "working the negative": bringing your legs into a pike position (both legs straight and close together) as you lower down as slowly as you possibly can!

Pike Press

Of all the handstand variations in this book, for me, the pike press was the most challenging variation to learn. Likely because I wasn't able to use my hip flexibility as much to come up, and the longer lever (the straight legs) required me to recruit a lot more upper-body strength as the load of my legs (in this case, the amount of weight I needed to lift without any momentum) increased once I straightened them. While I do have a good amount of hamstring flexibility, I'm also a runner and cyclist, and some days, my quads and hamstrings *feel* pretty tight, adding to the challenge.

What helped? Practicing at least one of the previous press variations and/or drills for a few minutes each day in my yoga practice until I felt ready to give it a go.

———

If you, too, feel ready to try a pike press, set up just as you did the previous presses, with your feet close together. Exactly how close depends on what feels best in your body. You could start with hip-width apart and then narrow or widen your stance as you like.

Shift your weight forward and push the floor away as you rise up onto your toes.

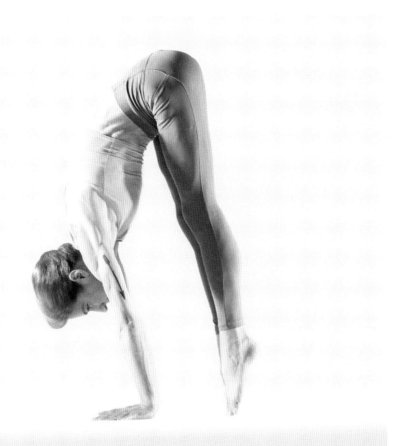

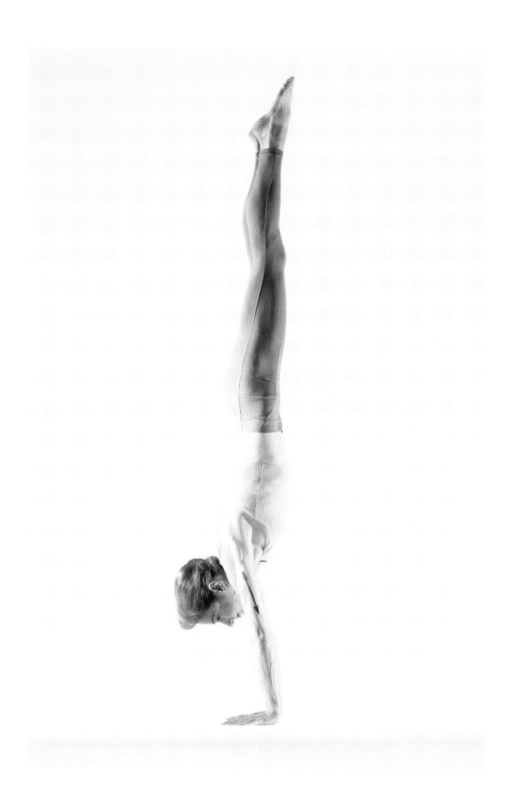

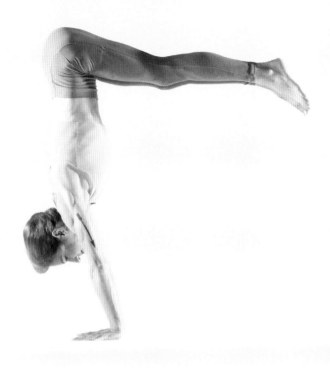

When your toes float up, keep your legs straight behind you (as opposed to straddling your legs or bending your knees as you come up), driving your hips over your shoulders.

Perhaps you keep going until you straighten your legs completely!

You can pike your legs all the way down, "working the negative" to come out, or exit any other way you like.

INCORPORATING HANDSTANDS INTO A SUN SALUTATION: WHAT TO PRACTICE

There are lots of ways to incorporate handstanding into a sun salute or vinyasa flow, from "hop switching" your legs in the air and landing your nonhopping foot at the top of your mat in warrior I in sun salute B, to jumping into a handstand before landing at the top of your mat in a forward bend, to "floating forward" (more on that on page 88), to anything else you can imagine!

Here's a drill you can practice to gain the skills and confidence you'll need. In particular, I love this one because it's accessible to a variety of handstand-experience levels: you can customize it by making the hops as big or as small as you like. It's also great for getting your heart rate up and, frankly, I think it's a whole lot of fun!

Downward-Facing-Dog Hop Switches

From a short downward-facing dog with feet close together:

Inhale, lift your left leg in the air, rise up onto the ball of your right foot, and gaze forward.

Exhale, bend your right knee and hop off of your right foot, then switch your legs in the air so you land on your left foot with the left knee bent.

Repeat, hopping off your left foot this time and switching your legs to land on your right foot.

Continue for a few more rounds. (I'll often set a timer for thirty seconds when I practice these.)

Tip: Start out with small hop switches, staying pretty low to the ground. Over time, you can make them bigger if you like, gradually working your hips higher and maybe even catching a little handstand hang time before you switch!

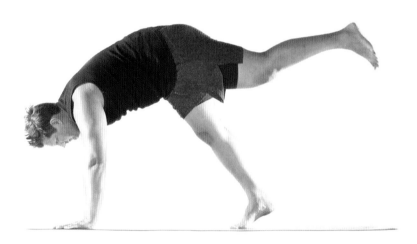

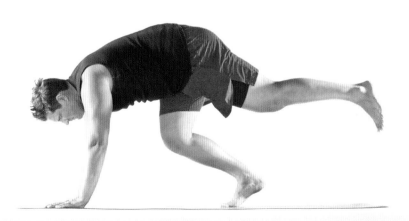

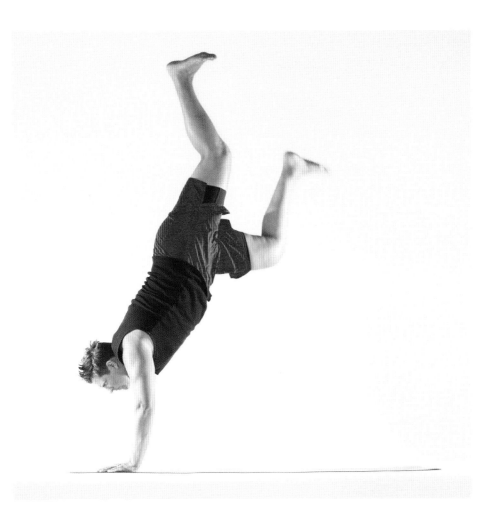

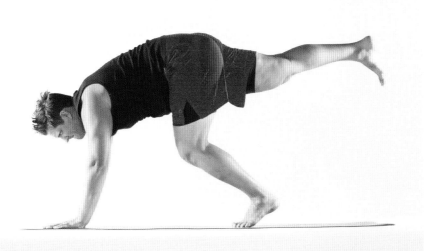

Floating Forward to Forward Bend from Downward-Facing Dog (Incorporating a "Handstand Hover")

Have you ever heard your yoga teacher give the option to "step, jump, or float forward" into a standing forward bend from downward-facing dog and wondered what the heck they were talking about? I know I have. What's the difference between a "float" and a "jump" anyway? It took me a while—over a decade of hearing this cue—before I figured it out. And here's the differentiation that finally made it click:

When you jump forward, you land on both feet pretty much right away, but when you float forward, you hover (in a position similar to the one you would be in if you were pressing into handstand and both feet just came up off of the ground) for a moment or two and then lower down with control.

Here's how to do it:

Start in a short downward-facing dog. I like to have my feet close together, but some folks prefer a wider stance.

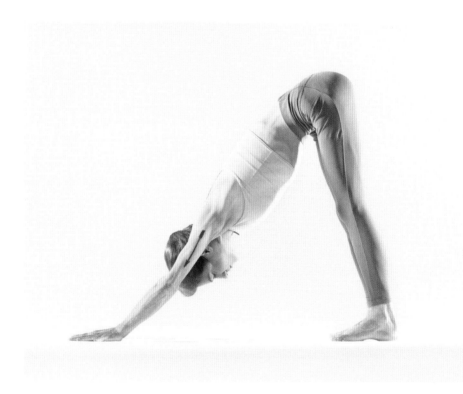

Inhale, rise up onto the balls of your feet, and gaze toward your hands.
Exhale, bend your knees, keep your heels lifted, and . . .

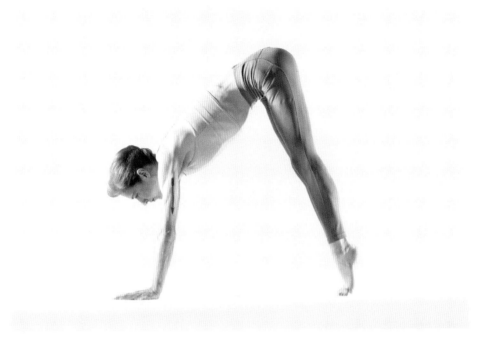

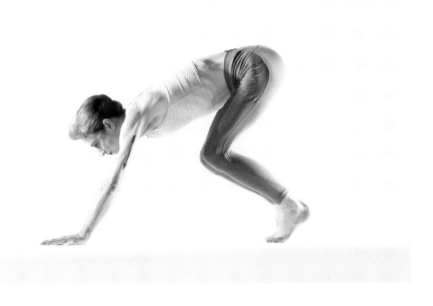

Jump off both feet, bringing your hips up over your shoulders.

Press a lot of weight into your fingertips and aim to hover in the handstand. Then slowly, with control, begin to lower your feet to the ground, perhaps hovering them just above the floor for a moment, maybe even tapping your toes to your wrists!

Then lower both feet together to land in a forward bend.

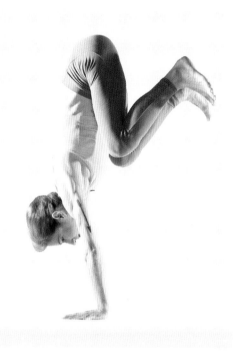

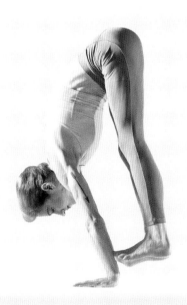

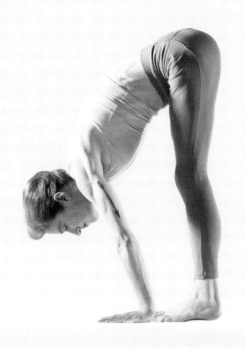

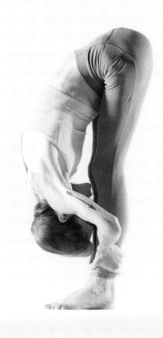

Tips for Happy Wrists and Forearms

Feel like your wrists and forearms could use a little love after all that handstanding? I got you covered. Try one or all of these variations to find some relief.

1. Wrist reliever: Sit, kneel, or stand in a comfortable position. With your left hand, grasp your right wrist. (For me, the sweet spot is just below the heel of my hand.) Squeeze your wrist and, keeping that, pull forward, like you were trying to draw your hand away from your elbow. Hold for a few breaths, then release and change sides. You can also do this wrist reliever periodically between handstands, planks, vinyasa flows, downward-facing dogs, or any time your wrists need some attention.

2. Forearm squeeze in lizard lunge: Shout out to model Nam, who taught me this one on set, during the photo shoot for this book! (Demonstrated here by Kyle, who is a video editor and often has weary wrists and forearms.)

In a wide lunge, with your right foot forward, tuck your right forearm nice and snug under your right knee, palm facing up. You get to control the pressure here; squeeze as strongly or as softly as you like. Feel free to adjust the position of your forearm, squeezing in different places, perhaps holding for a little longer anywhere that feels particularly good. Stay for a few breaths, then change sides.

3. Forearm squeeze in a squat: You can also do the previous exercise on both sides at the same time, approaching it from a squat instead of a lunge.

4. Self-massage for wrists and forearms: From hands and knees, bend your right elbow and turn your palm to face up, placing your right forearm on the floor in a place that feels comfortable and accessible to you. Use either of your knees (whichever one feels most natural for you) to apply light pressure on the soft tissue of your wrist and forearm. Gradually use your knee to massage all the way up to the place just below your elbow, and then work your way back down again. Feel free to hold at any place that feels particularly good. Here, too, you control the pressure. To increase the pressure, lift the foot of your massaging leg off of the floor.

Adjust your position as needed so that you're comfortable. For example, sometimes I like to place a block under my forehead as I do this, to allow my head and neck to relax.

Give yourself the gift of this massage for a minute or two before changing sides.

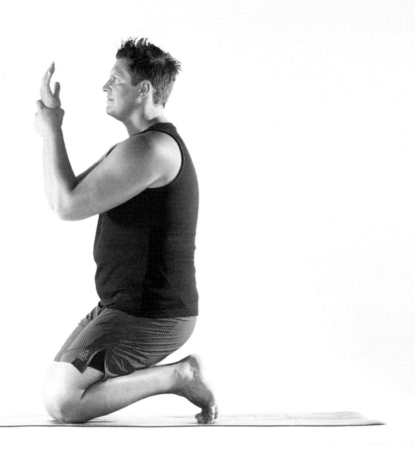

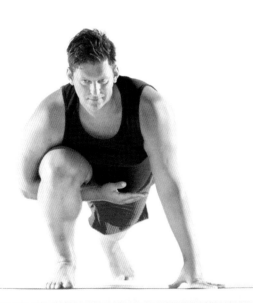

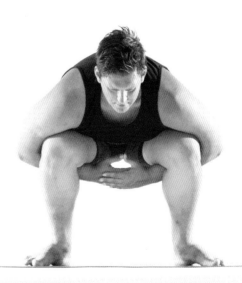

Forearm Stand

(Pincha Mayurasana)

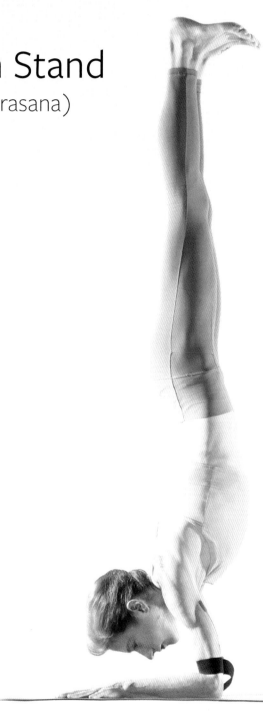

Literally "peacock tailfeather pose" in Sanskrit (pincha mayurasana, often nicknamed just pincha), forearm stand will always hold a special place in my heart.

The process of learning it helped me to gain confidence during an especially challenging time in my life. I had just gone through a divorce after moving across the country a couple of years prior. I was in school but at a loss about what I actually wanted to study or if I could even afford to continue. Yoga was my refuge, but I was also burned out from teaching over twenty classes a week (not counting teacher trainings, workshops, and private lessons). And did I mention that I also had a stressful retail job and was moonlighting as a freelance writer? I needed a bright spot, something fun to focus on. (Along with, it goes without saying, a good night's sleep!)

One day, while taking a class with the owner (a very skilled yoga teacher and therapist) of a studio where I taught, we did a "headless handstand" variation similar to the one on page 105. I had done forearm stand in its traditional form (forearms parallel with a little bit of a backbend), and I'd been able to hover my feet away from the wall for a second or two, but it wasn't until I tried this variation, which gave me a more stable base and didn't require the backbend, that I thought, "Hey, maybe I can learn to do this thing in the middle of the room someday . . ." So I made that a fun goal: I would practice forearm-balance variations at and away from the wall and see if I could eventually do one freestanding! This was also right around the time Instagram was brand-new, so I began to follow other arm-balance enthusiasts, pick up tips and tricks to try, and then tweak them to make them work for me.

As to not add more to my already too-full schedule, I would practice in the studio before students arrived to my daily classes. Thanks to Portland, Oregon's less-than-ideal bus schedule, I would usually end up arriving quite a bit early, so figured I should make the most of my time. Throughout the process I learned a lot (and eventually reached my goal!), much of which I've condensed in this chapter to share with you and to perhaps save you much of the trial and error I went through figuring it out.

A lot of the tips and variations I picked up from others were helpful but not always ideal for my body and proportions, so I adjusted accordingly. And later, when teaching pincha mayurasana variations to others and helping them build custom plans of their own, I realized that the things that worked for me didn't necessarily work for them, which taught me how to adapt accordingly! For example, I learned that my long-limbed friends often had a harder time getting their hips up over their shoulders to come into the variations, particularly if they also have shorter torsos.

As we explore these variations below, I encourage you to take a similar curious approach (while hopefully *not* burning the candle at both ends as I was—trust me when I say that my inversion and yoga practice overall leveled up significantly after I eventually started getting enough sleep and was able to take days off, a privilege I do not take for granted and that I believe everyone should have). While I try to include a variety of variations, tips, and approaches here, there are myriad other approaches, too, and many left to be discovered. Maybe you'll discover some along the way! Because you know your body a whole lot better than I do, and the purpose of this chapter and this book is not to tell you what to do but offer you resources and tools to customize forearm stand just for you so that you can enjoy it as much as I now do and use the process of figuring it out as a way to love, celebrate, and enjoy your uniqueness.

BENEFITS OF FOREARM STAND

Pincha, along with its preps and drills, requires and thus builds shoulder, back, and core strength. As with many inversions, many folks, me included, say it helps them to feel energized and refreshed, sometimes quite literally flipping their perspective when needed. It can also increase circulation. In addition, forearm stand requires a lot of focus and balance and thus enhances those as you work toward and practice it.

It also helps build crucial skills for other inversions. Your experience may differ, but I found that after learning to balance in forearm stand, balancing in handstand and headstand became a lot easier. And learning to balance on your forearms with your head off the floor in pincha can also help you to bring less weight into your head and neck in headstand.

GENERAL CAUTIONS AND CONTRAINDICATIONS

Shoulder or spinal injuries or recent surgeries, untreated high blood pressure, and glaucoma or other conditions where you need to avoid pressure in the eyes are considered contraindicated for forearm stand. As always, check with a qualified medical professional before trying anything you're unsure about.

Plank Walks

Purpose: To increase shoulder, back, and core strength; to build endurance; to practice and isolate the shoulder-over-elbow alignment that's key for pincha with parallel forearms.

In Practice: Begin in plank with knees lifted, like Shanté, or with your knees on the ground. Take a breath cycle here, then on your next inhale, lower your right forearm, stacking shoulder over elbow, followed by your left. Exhale, bring your right hand up first, then your left. Repeat, leading with your left this time, and then continue for thirty seconds, switching lead arms each time (down left, right; up left, right; down right, left; up right, left; etc.). This can be a brain teaser, but don't worry if you get your sides mixed up; it really doesn't matter! Just keep going if you get mixed up. As with meditation, noticing when your mind wanders and then bringing it back is all part of the practice and helps cultivate focus over time.

Try doing this drill two to four times total, resting for ten seconds in between rounds.

Tips: To up the endurance challenge, go faster! To focus on alignment, slow the drill down.

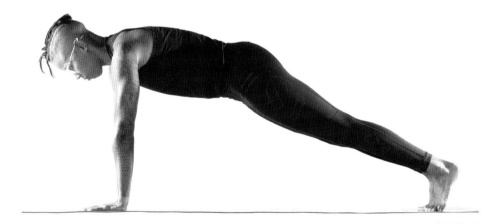

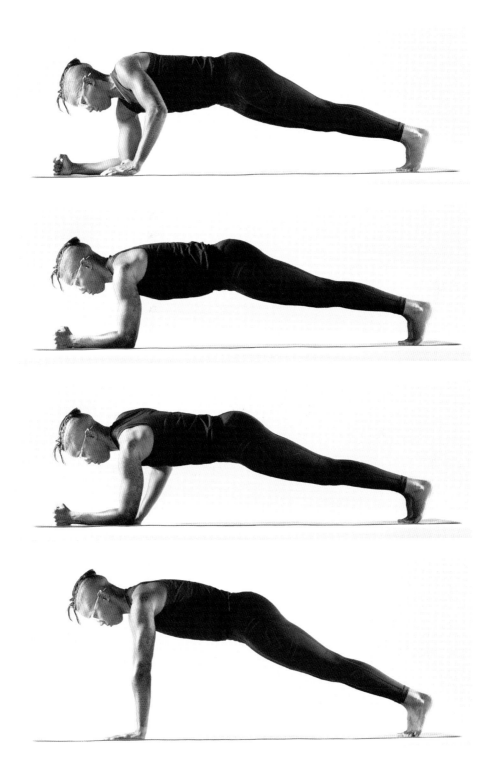

Tricep Presses

Purpose: Not gonna lie: these are killer. But they're also *effective* for helping you learn to keep your forearms hugging in so that your elbows don't splay in pincha. They also build tricep strength, back and shoulder strength, core strength, and *definitely* endurance!

In Practice: Start on forearms and knees with your knees a little behind your hips. Lift your elbows slightly off the ground and then begin to pulse them up and down without letting them touch the floor. Continue for thirty seconds, breathing in whatever way feels natural.

Aim for three to four rounds, resting for ten seconds between each.

I highly suggest doing these on your knees to start, as shown, but if you want to up the load and the challenge by doing them from knees-up plank, you do you.

You can also regress the drill (decreasing the load slightly) by doing these from table, with your knees under your hips.

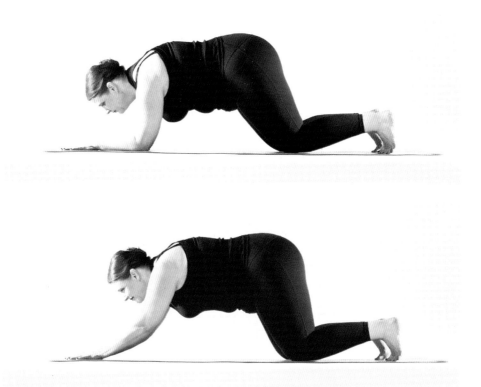

Forearm Side Plank

Purpose: To asymmetrically strengthen back and shoulder muscles, work on shoulder-over-elbow alignment, and work on balance.

In Practice: From forearm plank, begin to roll onto the outer edge of your right foot, adjusting your right forearm as needed so that it's in a comfortable position with your shoulder above or slightly behind your elbow—perhaps keeping it parallel with the long edges of the mat, like Sarah, which offers an additional balance challenge, or turning it in slightly so it's at about a forty-five-degree angle, which can make balancing easier. Keep your left fingertips on the floor for balance, or bring your left hand to your hip, or reach it up to the sky as you open into side plank.

You can do side plank kneeling, or with your right leg straight and your left knee bent and planted in front of your right like a kickstand; or you can stack your left leg on top of your right, or gradually work toward doing so, finding a midway position to hold, like Sarah.

Hold for fifteen seconds to start, then change sides, perhaps building to sixty seconds on each side over time.

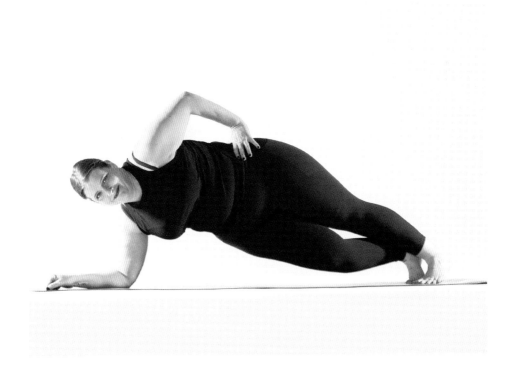

Reclined Hero Pose (*Supta Virasana*)

Purpose: To stretch your quads, hip flexors, abdomen, chest, and shoulders in order to make pincha easier to get into and to prepare for backbend-focused variations. I am a cyclist and runner with tight quads, so this is an essential daily stretch for me, and I always do it before practicing pincha mayurasana.

In Practice: From a high kneeling position, toes untucked, separate your feet wider than your hips and lower your seat toward the floor. (You can sit on a block or folded blanket if the floor feels far away.)

Arrange your feet so they're just outside your hips; the tops of your feet are on the floor and your toes are pointing straight back. If you're sitting on a prop, hug it with your feet and ankles and reach back through your big toes. This might be an intense enough stretch as is, but if not and you feel comfortable, begin to walk your palms back, resting your hands on the ground. (If you're sitting on a block, this is likely as far as you'll be able to go.) If you'd like to recline further, come onto your elbows, as I am demonstrating, or all the way onto your back—perhaps reaching your arms overhead and bringing the back of your hands to the floor. If you feel knee or other discomfort, back off and come more upright.

Stay for a minute or two, then press yourself upright and rise back up to high kneeling.

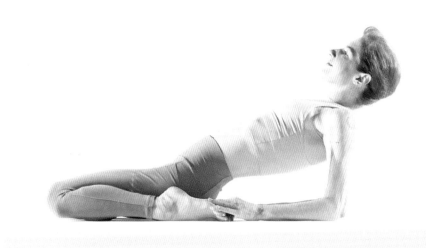

Revolved Lizard Lunge with Foot Grab

Purpose: To stretch your quads, hip flexors, chest, and shoulders one side at a time and to mobilize your spine.

In Practice: Come into a wide low lunge with your right foot forward, your right knee and toes pointing in the same direction, and both hands inside your right foot on the ground or blocks, left knee down, and left toes tucked.

Bring your right hand onto your right thigh. Inhale, lengthen your spine, and on an exhale, twist your torso to the right. Stay here or, for more of a hip-flexor stretch, draw your left heel in toward your seat. Grab the pinky-toe side of your left foot with your right hand.

Tip: If you prop up your left knee on a block and/or your left hand, this can make grabbing your foot easier. And if you're prone to hamstring cramps in the pose like me, I personally find that the addition of blocks keeps those at bay.

To intensify the stretch, bend your right elbow to draw your left heel in toward your glutes.

Stay for five to ten breaths and see if you can roll a little more onto the outer edge of your left knee (the back knee will tend to roll in).

To exit, on an inhale, release your back foot with control and untwist. Switch sides.

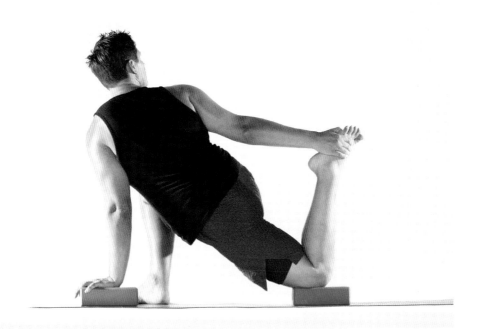

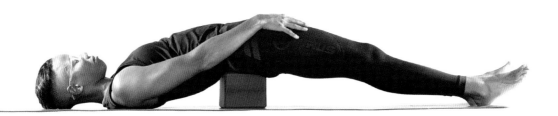

Hip-Flexor Stretch on Block

Purpose: To stretch the entire front of your body, especially your psoas, quads, and abdomen, and also your chest and shoulders.

In Practice: Lie on your back with your knees bent, feet on the floor about hip-width apart, knees and toes pointing in the same direction and heels under your knees or a little forward of them, arms alongside you, and a block within reach.

Make sure there's a little space between the back of your neck and the floor. Inhale, lift your pelvis and place the block underneath it at any height, adjusting as needed. (Avoid placing the block under your low back, which can become uncomfortable after holding the pose for a while.) Let your pelvis sink into the support of the block.

If this feels great, feel free to stay. To intensify the stretch, you can stretch your right leg out long, isolating the right side a bit. Keep your left foot on the floor or bend your left knee into your chest. To further intensify, reach your right arm up overhead. Stay for five to ten breaths, then return to supported bridge and change sides.

You can also stretch both sides at the same time, straightening both legs, like Shanté. Bring your hands to the fronts of your thighs, reach them overhead to intensify, or place them anywhere that feels good. Stay for five to ten breaths, then place your feet back on the floor, one at a time.

To come out, lift your hips, remove the block, and lower your pelvis.

Tip: Keeping your legs and feet in a neutral position (with your knees and tops of your feet pointing to the sky), as opposed to turned out, makes this more of a hip-flexor and quad stretch.

For any and all of the variations that follow, you can practice at or away from a wall.

I recommend starting at the wall, about a forearm's distance away, so that you have room to come up but are close enough to easily rest your heels on it.

You can gradually move away from the wall as your ability to balance with your heels off the wall grows, if and as you have an "exit strategy" you feel comfortable with if you lose your balance away from the wall.

I like cartwheeling one leg at a time off to the side if I lose my balance. If you're one of those lucky folks who's fine flipping over into viparita dandasana (a wheel pose, or big backbend, on your forearms), hey, go to town. When I was first learning forearm stands, I flipped over into a backbend a *lot*, which for me wasn't my favorite way to exit, but it wasn't awful either, as long as I adequately prepared my body for backbends. While I *did* start to feel much better in a viparita dandasana overall, I'm glad I discovered the cartwheel-out method soon after, as it feels more sustainable for me.

"Headless Headstand" with Prayer Hands

Start on all fours and lower to your forearms, stacking shoulders over elbows. Bring your hands into prayer, or clasp them if you prefer (tuck your bottom pinky in so not to crush it). Tuck your toes, lift your hips, and come into dolphin.

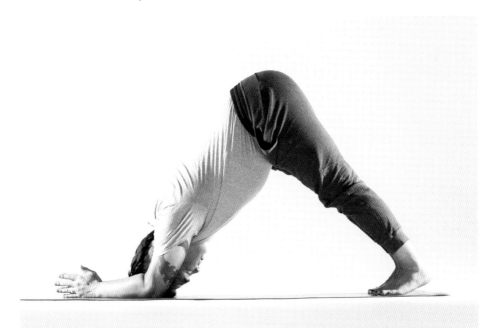

Forearm Stand (Pincha Mayurasana)

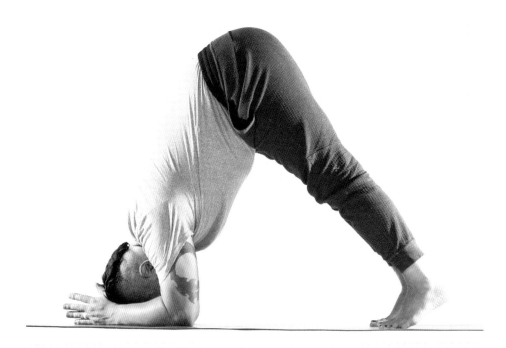

Walk your feet forward so that your shoulders are over your elbows and your hips are as close as you can get them to stacked over your shoulders. Gaze back toward your legs. Hug your forearms in and press the outer edges of your hands, wrists, and forearms firmly into the floor. Keep your head off the floor.

Inhale, lift your left leg high in the air (your hip can turn out) and rise onto the ball of your right foot.

Exhale, bend your right knee, and hop up into a forearm balance.

Keep hugging your forearms in and pressing them into the floor.

Tuck your chin slightly so your crown is facing (but not touching) the floor.

Aim to stay for about three to five breaths, then lower one leg at a time to come down. Repeat, lifting your left leg first this time.

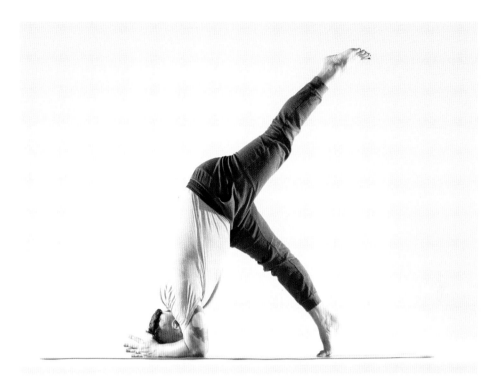

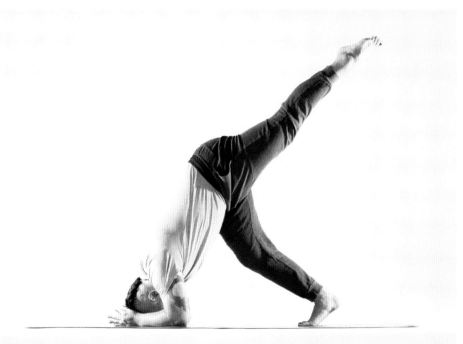

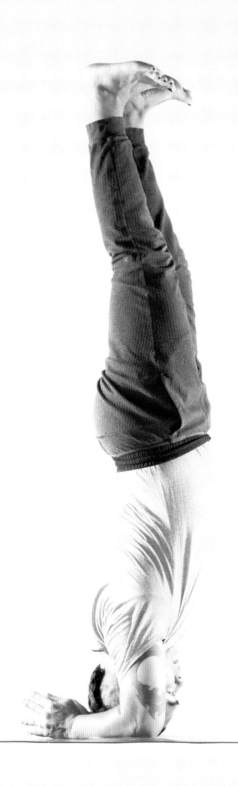

Tips: When you come up, take a moment to find your balance before bringing your legs together. It's usually a little easier to figure out if there's some space between your two legs, so taking a moment to get stable before your legs come together sets you up for success!

Instead of hopping, you can also press into this or any forearm-stand variation. We explore pressing more in chapters 3 (handstand) and 5 (headstand), but here are the basics for pressing into a forearm stand:

- As with hopping into it, from dolphin, walk your feet as close to your hands as possible without elbows splaying. Keep hugging your elbows in and pressing your forearms down.

- Lift your right leg high, opening your right hip, and rise up as high as you can onto your right toes. *Really* reach up with your left toes.

- Shift your shoulder forward, beyond your elbows, and push the ground away even more strongly as you continue to reach up with your left toes until maybe . . . your right toes float off the ground!

- If they do, once you find your balance (spreading your toes can help), bring your right leg to meet your left.

Here, too, lower one foot at a time to come down, then switch sides.

Pincha Mayurasana ("Peacock Tailfeather Pose") Variations

You'll come into these similarly to how you approached headless headstand. Start in dolphin, but this time with your forearms parallel to each other, palms down.

Tip: Remember, keeping your forearms parallel but turning your hands out can keep the elbow splay at bay!

Walk your feet forward as much as possible while keeping forearms parallel. Gaze toward your hands and on an inhale, lift your left leg high and rise up onto your right toes. On an exhale, hop (or press) up into pincha, keeping your gaze toward your hands. If you find your balance, bring your left leg to meet your right.

You'll likely notice that this variation is more of a backbend than headless headstand and requires more shoulder mobility.

Stay for three to five breaths, then lower one leg at a time to come down. Repeat, lifting your right leg first.

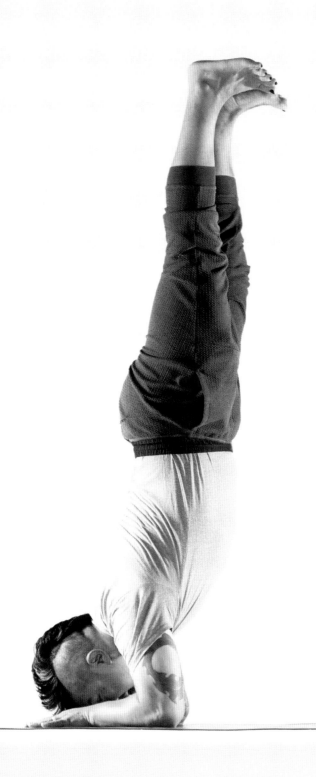

Forearm Stand Holding a Block

Holding a block between your hands is a great way to keep your elbows from splaying. Hold the block on its flattest, widest setting. Actually grip it with your hands so that your fingers and thumbs wrap around it. If you have broad shoulders, you might prefer two blocks placed next to each other.

If you're feeling strong in your forearm stands and want to add a new challenge, try practicing with palms facing up instead of down. This requires more shoulder rotation than usual, so I use a block to give me a boundary to push into, which not only keeps my elbows in but also helps me to feel more balanced and engaged overall. For this variation, instead of holding the block, I place it between my hands and press the pinky edges into it as I spin my thumbs down toward the ground.

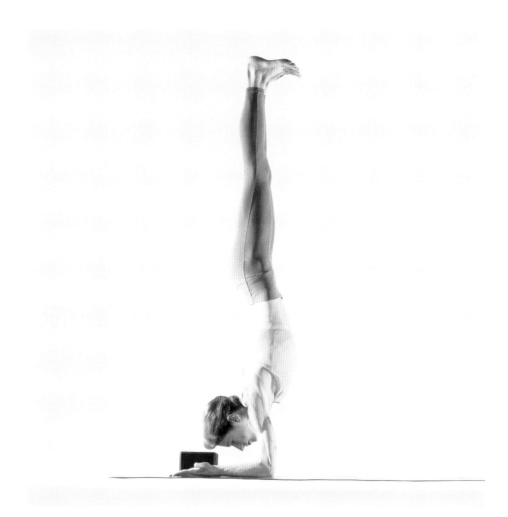

Forearm Stand with a Strap

While some find hugging in while holding a block to be most useful, others prefer to keep their elbows in by looping a strap snuggly around their upper arms and pushing out against it. Make a loop that's about your shoulder-width apart, then cinch the strap around your upper arms just above your elbows, loose enough so that you can still place your forearms on the ground to come into pincha with your elbows right under your shoulders but taught enough so that when you push out against the strap your elbows don't move.

This option and the option to hug into a block both utilize an isometric contraction—a muscle contraction that doesn't change the angle of a joint (i.e., result in movement) but instead is used to stabilize.

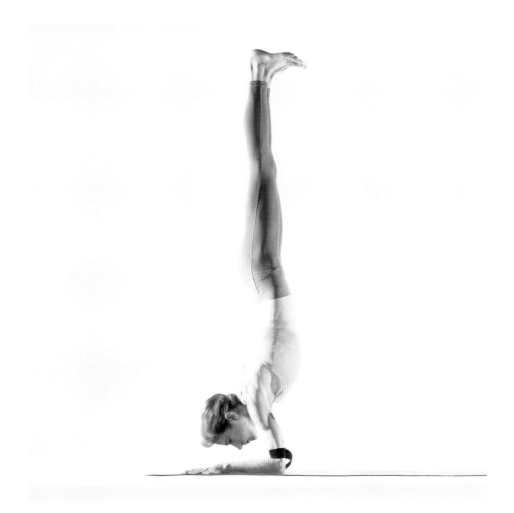

Hollowback Forearm Stands

I can't be the only one who sees "hollowback" and immediately starts singing Gwen Stefani's "Hollaback Girl," right?

And it is kind of fitting, because when you see these variations depicted for the first time, if you're anything like me, "This shit is bananas . . ." might be your first thought.

But if you're looking for an interesting way to change up your forearm stands, these backbendy balances might be just the thing to spice up your practice. It can also be a nice prep scorpion pose (vrschikasana), a backbend-forearm stand hybrid that Dianne Bondy and I break down in *Yoga Where You Are.*

I highly recommend starting at the wall, and make sure you're confident practicing headless headstand on forearms. (A hollowback is basically a headless headstand plus a backbend, only instead of opening your chest toward your hands, you're pushing it back between your arms in the opposite direction.)

Set up for headless headstand with prayer hands (page 105) quite close to the wall: fingers almost touching.

If you find later that you want a deeper backbend, you can set up a little farther away next time.

Come into dolphin, walk your feet toward your hands, and come up into headless headstand with both heels on the wall. Continue to hug your elbows in and push into the floor, and tuck your chin slightly so that you're looking into the room behind you (not at the wall that your heels are on). Flex your feet and press the backs of your thighs into (or toward) the wall. Keep your low belly engaged: squeeze your two front hip "points" (anterior superior iliac spines, or ASIS for the anatomy geeks) toward each other like you're cinching a drawstring, squeeze your pubic bone toward your navel as though zipping a zipper between them, and continue to push the ground away so that your low back and shoulders don't have to do quite so much work.

Maintain that power and engagement as you press your chest farther back through your arms, away from the wall, and reach up through your inner heels.

Stay for a few breaths, and lower one leg at a time to come down.

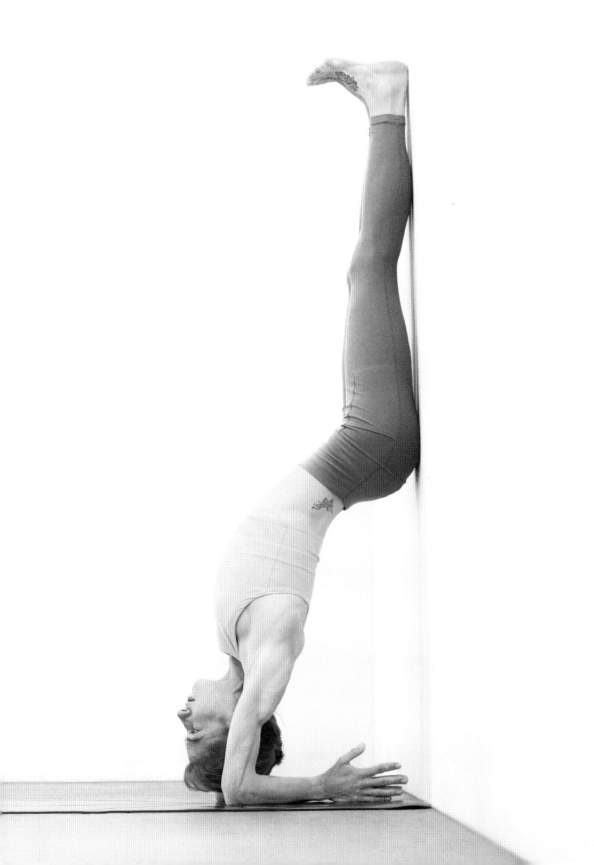

Variations and Progression

In lieu of stag legs (pictured and described below), you can keep both legs straight, like the splits upside down.

If you feel ready to try hollowback in the middle of the room, make sure you have an exit strategy you're confident with and start with a legs-apart version like stag legs or splits.

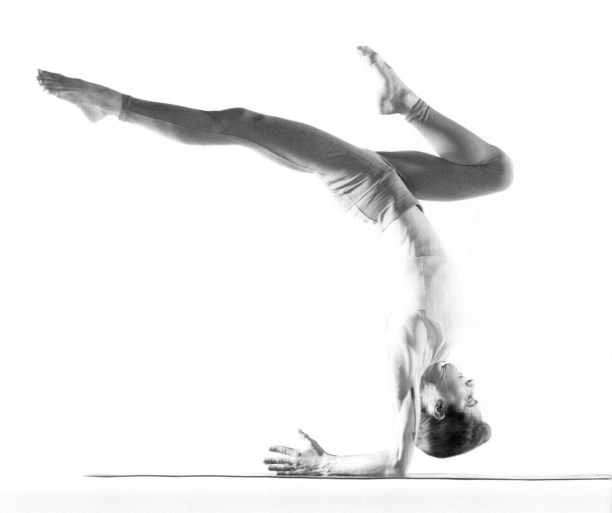

With Stag Legs

This variation is a great place to start if you're interested in taking hollowback off the wall. Remember: split legs make it easier to find your balance!

———

Bring the short edge of your mat to the wall and set up for headless headstand with hands in prayer, facing the wall, with your fingers a little closer than a leg's length away from it. The exact distance differs for us all depending on our proportions, but err on the side of being just a little closer to the wall than necessary so you're confident your foot can connect with it. You can always come down and adjust if you're too close.

Press up into dolphin, walk your feet toward your hands, and lift your left leg high in the air, rising up onto your right toes to hop or press up with your legs apart. Bring the ball of your left foot to connect with the wall. Keep your left leg straight and bend your right knee to make "stag legs" (which resemble a deer leaping through the air).

Resist your elbows in and push the ground away. Press the ball of your right foot into the wall as you reach your left knee away from it and press your chest back through your arms, keeping your chin tucked slightly as your crown hovers from the floor.

To come out, push off the wall with your left foot and lower your left foot to the floor (behind you) first, followed by your right. Repeat on the other side.

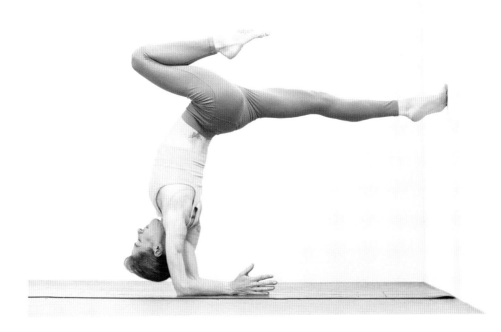

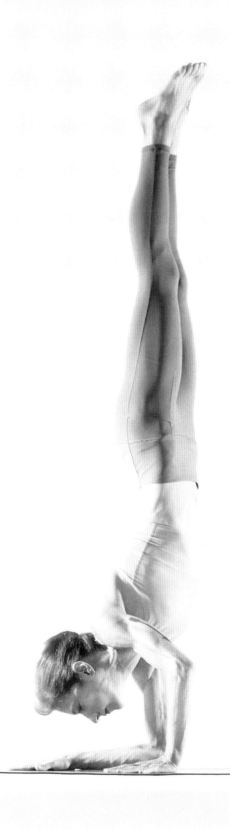

Asymmetrical Forearm Stand ("Funky Pincha")

Though this is often considered a more challenging option, I usually have an easier time coming up into an asymmetrical forearm stand than a symmetrical one (particularly when my shoulders feel tight), reminding me once more how unique our bodies and experiences really are.

You can think of this as a forearm stand-handstand hybrid.

―――――

Start on hands and knees and lower onto your right forearm, shoulder over elbow.

Walk your left hand back so that your left wrist is in line with your right elbow.

This is my preferred starting place, but others prefer to start with their left hand farther back, so that their left fingertips are in line with their right elbow. Try both ways to see which feels best for you.

Hug your left elbow in toward you (think "chaturanga arms"), tuck your toes under, and lift your knees to press up into a dolphin–downward-facing-dog hybrid. Walk your feet forward as in the other variations we explored, gazing slightly forward.

Inhale, lift your left leg high in the air and rise up onto the ball of your right foot. Exhale, hop or press up, keeping your legs apart while you find your balance. If you feel stable, bring your legs up and together. Keep pushing the ground away and hugging your left elbow in as you reach up through your heels.

Lower one foot at a time to come down, then repeat on the other side.

SAMPLE ONE-MONTH PLAN FOR LEARNING FOREARM STAND

- Choose any three days each week to do these practices every week for one month.

- Swap out drills and stretches as needed to best align with your needs and goals!

- Due to the similarities, this plan can also be used and adapted for headstand. See "Incorporating Headstand in Practice" on page 145 for details.

See "Learning Forearm Stand" tables in appendix 1 starting on page 182.

Headstand

(Sirsasana)

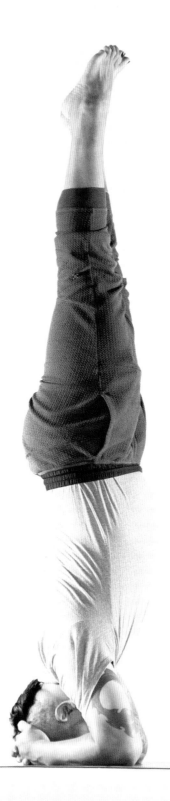

Though she may not have been the first to say it, one of my very first teachers, Karina Mirsky, once said something akin to "Yoga is less about standing on your head than it is about learning to stand strong in who you are."

And yes! I completely agree. You can absolutely practice—and more importantly *live*—your yoga without ever standing on your head. But learning to stand on your head can also be a fun, empowering challenge, and in this chapter we'll explore lots of ways to approach headstand and make it work for you.

BENEFITS

If you google "benefits of headstand," you'll get a long list of claims for the pose often dubbed "king of asanas."

Some of these are dubious, of course. Like headstand is *probably* not going to "reverse the flow of blood to your brain" because, you know that whole blood-brain barrier thing our bodies have going on. Or how about "alleviate depression"? Um. Wow. I will say that sometimes when I'm feeling down, going upside down shifts my perspective and can sometimes help me feel a little better. But pretty much any kind of joyful movement does that for me, and standing on my head is definitely no substitute for appropriate medical care. "Activates the pituitary and pineal glands"? That sounds good, but there is no credible evidence I could find to support this. "Flush out the adrenal glands"? Um, I don't think they work that way.

Other benefits, however, are a little more, um, *real*. (Or they can be for some people, some of the time.) For example:

"Stimulate the lymphatic system" and "decrease fluid buildup in the legs, ankles, and feet"? Absolutely! All movement is good for this, but unlike some tree frogs (fun fact), humans don't have a "lymph heart" to move lymphatic fluid through our bodies. In order to keep those juices pumpin', we have to move, and because we spend so much time in an upright position, going upside down is an especially efficient way to shake things up.

"Increase focus?" Sure! Inversions like headstand require a lot of focus to get into and hold, and that will naturally help to build our "focus muscles" (though I'm not going to stop taking my ADHD medicine anytime soon).

"Strengthen the upper body, spine, and core"? Yes! I wouldn't recommend inversions as your sole strength-building practice, but like other "active" inversions (handstand and forearm stand), handstand requires and builds strength in these areas.

I could go on, but if I tried to unpack all of the purported benefits of sirsasana, I would well exceed my allotted word count for this book, in this intro alone.

So if most inversions have the same benefits, why choose a headstand over one with a better rep (see "Why Headstand Gets a Bad Rap" on page 123)?

For one, it's easier for most of us to hold a headstand longer than handstand and forearm stand, which are typically harder to hold our balance in.

And even though headstand is considered "riskier" than handstand and forearm balance, it's easier for a lot of folks to get into, making it a more attractive, less intimidating option for many practitioners.

That said, for some of us, bearing weight on our heads is contraindicated. Luckily (come on, you knew this was coming!) there's a solution: Don't put your body at risk for the sake of a pose. No asana, even the "king," is worth that. Instead, adapt the pose to make it work for you.

In this chapter we'll look at preps and drills for headstand and explore how to approach the more traditional variations. We'll also look at variations that provide many of the same benefits but don't involve weight-bearing through your head and neck.

GENERAL CONTRAINDICATIONS

Head, neck, shoulder, and spinal injuries or recent surgeries (though for some people with neck or shoulder issues, variations that don't bear weight on those areas may be fine), untreated high blood pressure, glaucoma, or any condition where you need to avoid pressure on the eyes are considered contraindicated for headstand. Again, if you're unsure, check with your health-care provider before trying any pose or variation.

Why Headstand Gets a Bad Rap

In recent years, headstand has developed a reputation, and not a good one. Headstand (and shoulderstand) are often said to be "dangerous," and some yoga studios have even banned teachers from teaching them and students from practicing them within their walls. While I don't think anyone ever "needs" to do headstand, and I used to be on "team ban sirsasana!" myself, I no longer feel this way.

Why? I don't think it's wise to instill fear of movement in our students. There's something called the nocebo effect, which is basically the opposite of the placebo effect. Essentially this means that when we prime students for a negative outcome (e.g., "Headstand is injurious" or "You can seriously injure yourself in shoulderstand"), a negative outcome is actually more likely to occur. If we set the expectation that headstand—a movement that many bodies are able to do or, over time, build the capacity to do—could hurt someone, if they do at some point decide to try it, they're actually more likely to get hurt!

That doesn't mean teachers should open a beginning yoga class with headstand, or assume that everyone can and should do one, or that it doesn't matter how they do it.

It does mean, though, that if headstand is *not* contraindicated and someone *does* wish to learn it, that they can, over time, work with preps, drills, and variations that gradually increase the amount of load (weight-bearing) through the arms, shoulders, head, and neck to train their body to do a safe and sustainable headstand (same goes for shoulderstand too).

The bottom line? Listen to your body, check with your medical providers (yoga teachers and even yoga therapists are not medical providers), and if headstand is not contraindicated for you and you'd like to practice it, there's nothing "wrong" with working toward it. Doing so will ultimately make your tissues more "robust."

That said, contraindicated or not, if you're not interested in practicing or teaching headstand, no one says you have to.

(For a whole lot more info on the biomechanics of headstand and how to prepare for this pose, I highly recommend Jules Mitchell's book *Yoga Biomechanics* and Bernie Clark's *Your Body, Your Yoga* series.)

Sewing Machine Drills

Purpose: This drill is a classic for a reason! It's both a prep for and an alternative to headstand, and it helps to strengthen and mobilize your shoulders, both of which will help you cultivate a stable, sustainable headstand.

In Practice: Begin in dolphin pose (page 23) with hands interlaced (bottom pinky tucked in so you don't crush it) or in prayer.

On an inhale, shift forward, as though you were coming into a forearm plank, but (as long as it feels good for your shoulders) continue to shift forward so that your shoulders come past your elbows. You might briefly tap your nose on the floor in front of your hands if you can.

Do this for thirty seconds or about eight to ten reps.

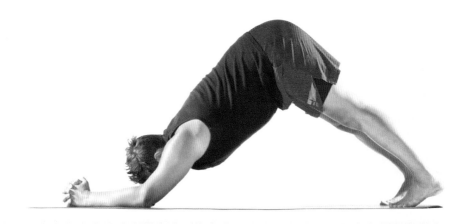

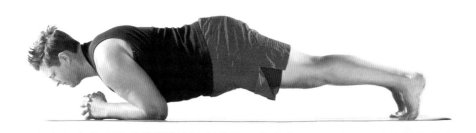

Headstand Prep Pressing Head into the Wall While Standing

Purpose: To get a felt sense of pressing your head against a surface, actively lengthening your spine, while remaining "right side up."

In Practice: Stand facing a wall in a wide stance and place your hands on it, a little wider than your shoulders. Place the crown of your head on the wall between your hands, then adjust your position—how far back your feet are and how low on the wall your hands are—until your spine is long and neutral (not rounding). Press your head into the wall and breathe here. As you press into the wall, envision your spine getting longer; instead of collapsing into your shoulders, neck, and head, you're lengthening out from them, similar to headstand, where you'll press against the floor to lift away from it as opposed to collapsing all of your weight into it.

Stay for three to five breaths, then gently release.

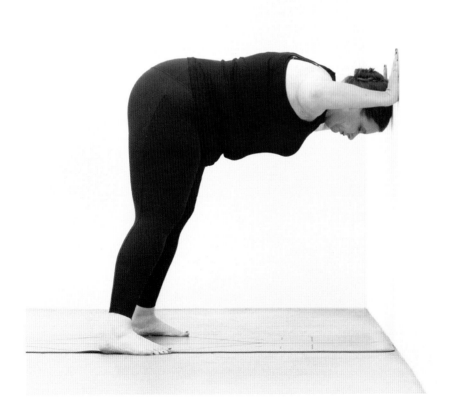

Yin Butterfly with Head on Block

Purpose: For some people, pressing their head into something firm (such as the floor in headstand or the wall in the previous variation) can be especially calming and grounding, but not everyone is able to (or wants to) go upside down. While it's your forehead pressing into the support here (as opposed to your crown), you may still find that this variation provides a similar sense of grounding. And if you are working toward a headstand, the hip-opening butterfly might make coming into it a little easier when practiced regularly and/or before your headstand.

In Practice: Sit on your mat in a long butterfly position, with feet farther away from your pelvis than they would be for a bound angle pose (baddha konasana). In yin yoga, this shape is called "butterfly," and in other styles of yoga, it's often called diamond pose (tarasana).

Begin sitting upright, and if your lower back rounds, try elevating your seat on a folded blanket or two and/or propping your feet up on a yoga block.

Have a separate yoga block nearby to support your head. Inhale, lengthen your spine, and on an exhale, begin to fold forward, allowing your spine to round. Place your nearby block at whatever height is appropriate for you in a position that will support your forehead, in whatever place makes sense for your proportions—perhaps on your feet, as Sarah is showing in the photo. Rest your arms and hands in any position that's comfortable for you.

Stay for one to two minutes, adjusting your block if needed and enjoying the gentle pressure against your forehead.

Tip: If the block isn't cutting it, you can place another prop, such as a bolster or folded blanket, under your forehead or you can stack a couple of blocks on top of each other.

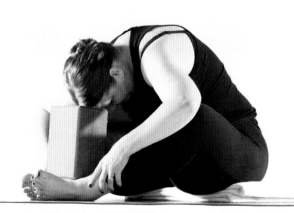

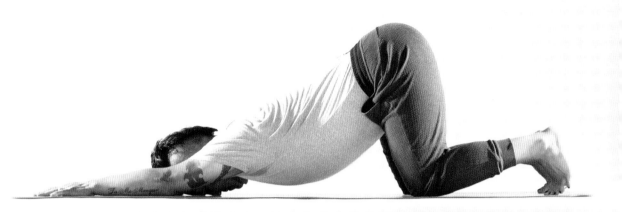

Puppy Pose

Purpose: To stretch, open, and prepare your shoulders and upper back for head-stand variations and experience the grounding support of your head (in this case again, your forehead) connecting with the earth.

In Practice: Begin on hands and knees and then walk your hands forward toward the top of your mat. Walk your knees back as needed so that your hips remain stacked roughly over them in the pose, and rest your forehead on the ground or a block or other prop. Focus on lengthening your spine as you relax your chest toward the floor. Externally rotate your upper arms, lifting your inner armpits up, in order to find more space through your neck and shoulders. For a more "active" version, come up onto your fingertips.

Stay for one to two minutes.

Note: This can be a great option for pregnant folks looking for an inversion alternative (especially ones like headstand that tend to be held for longer), and it also can be a nice alternative to downward-facing dog or child's pose too!

These variations allow you to experience the benefits of headstand without bearing weight through your head and neck.

They're also great skill-builders for the "traditional" weight-bearing variations of sirsasana and for forearm stand.

With Two Chairs and a Wall

Have you seen those inversion benches that seem to be the rage? They are no doubt an excellent option for a lot of people, but they can also set you back about $150 or so. If you have a couple of folding chairs, some blankets, and a wall available, this variation can be a more economical option!

———

Bring your mat to the wall for traction. (In the photo, Nam has his mat perpendicular to the wall, but for extra grip to keep your chairs solidly in place, place the mat parallel against the wall so that all four legs of each chair can be on it.)

You'll need two chairs of equal height for this one, and you can use yoga chairs if you have them (which are folding chairs with the backrests removed), but standard folding chairs work fine.

Bring the chairs all the way against the wall with the seats facing each other. Their exact distance depends on your proportions: you'll need enough space for your head to fit between them as one chair supports each shoulder. Place a folded blanket (or folded yoga mat) on each chair seat for cushioning and support. You can also place a folded sticky mat under each blanket (with the folded mat's edges in line with the edge of the chair seat) to keep the blankets from sliding. You'll also want the mats and/or blankets you use to be the same thickness so that the height of your support is even on both sides.

Come onto your knees in front of your setup, facing the wall. Place your head between the two chairs so that your shoulders are supported by the blankets and/or mats and about two-thirds of the way toward the wall.

From there, grip the outside edges of the chairs with each hand, with your thumbs under the blankets/mats and your fingers under the seats.

Tuck your toes under, lift your knees away from the floor and walk your feet toward the wall until you can tuck your knees into your chest and bring your legs up the wall.

You can keep your arms and hands as they are, in a position similar to chaturanga, or, if you feel super stable and comfortable here, like Nam, you can slide one arm at a time through each chairback, palms facing up or down.

Keep your gaze relaxed and allow your head to hang freely. Your heels will remain on the wall the whole time, but try to keep your hips off the wall.

Stay as long as you like (several breaths, even a minute or two). When you're ready to come down, if they're not already there, return one arm at a time to its starting chaturanga-like position, gripping the chair seat, and lower down with control in the reverse order that you came up.

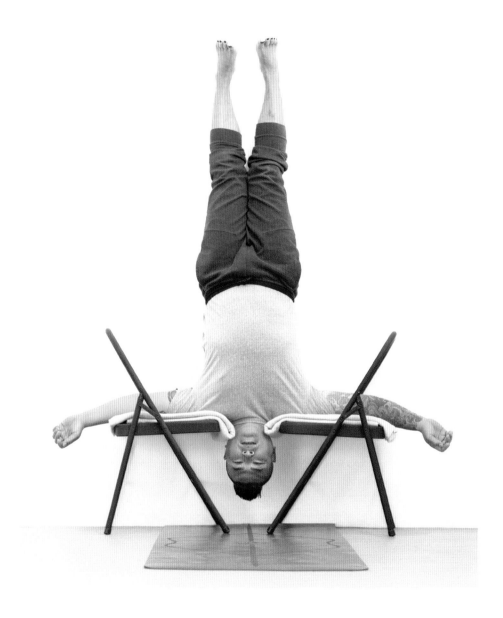

With Blocks at the Wall

You can do a similar variation using blocks. For this one, you can set up your mat perpendicular to the wall. Take three blocks, on their lowest setting, and line them up in a row with their long edges touching each other and the short edges flush against the wall. Then slide out the middle block and set it aside. The two remaining blocks are the first blocks in your stacks. The middle block you moved aside was used to measure the right amount of space for your head. From there, you can add to your stacks!

For a lot of people, three thicker blocks on each side or four thinner blocks on each side is a good starting place, but depending on your proportions, you may need to add or remove blocks. The key is to make sure that your height is even on both sides and that the crown of your head is able to hang above the floor in the pose without touching. It's okay if your hair touches the floor. Be sure that all of the blocks are flush against the wall.

———

Kneel in front of your setup, facing the wall, and plant your hands flat on the mat so that the tips of your longest fingers touch the bottom blocks. Bring your head between the blocks and your shoulders on top of them, scooting your upper back close to the wall.

Lift one leg up high in the air, opening your hip to give you some leverage. Keep reaching up through your top leg until your bottom leg floats away from the floor (try to avoid kicking up). If you're not quite able to get up, you can try the "tuck" method from the chair variation, or, if available, ask an experienced yoga teacher or qualified friend to give you a leg up. Press your hands strongly into the ground and allow your head to dangle.

Tip: If your palms don't touch the floor, come down one leg at a time and then re-enter the pose with some support under your hands to add height, such as a block under each hand on its lowest setting or a firm folded blanket under your hands, depending on how much height you need.

If your head is on the floor, come down and add a block to each stack. Remain in the pose for several breaths. (But come down before you feel like you "need" to!)

You can keep your legs extended on the wall, as Shanté is, or rest your feet on a chair seat as Peggy is. (Though I would recommend setting up the chair so that you can place your feet on the front of the seat instead of sliding them through the back, as Peggy is, to allow for an easier exit. Peggy is very familiar with this pose and has an alternative "escape route" she likes for this one, but most of us will find that an option where we can move our legs more freely is preferable.)

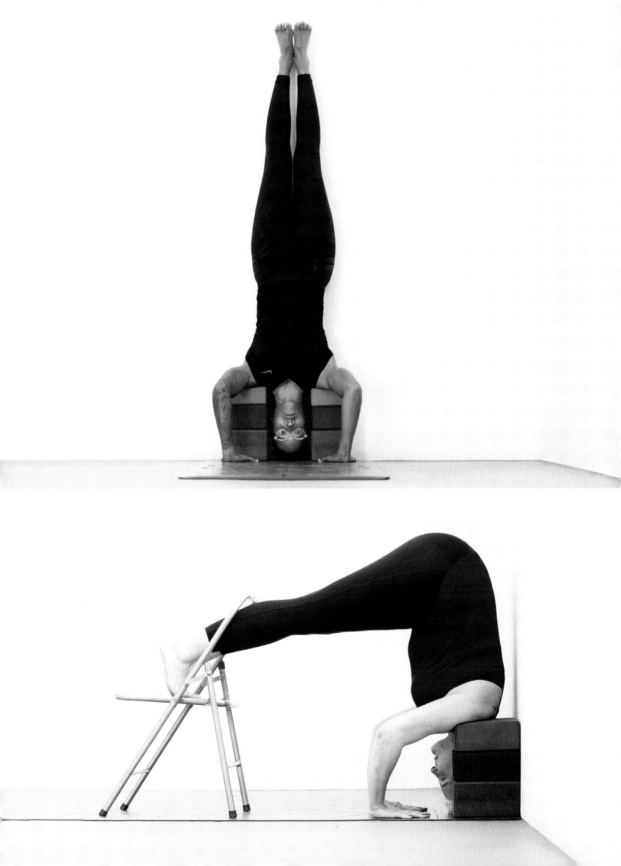

With "Stonehenge" Setup at the Wall

If you've read my previous book with Dianne Bondy, *Yoga Where You Are*, you might be familiar with this variation already. I like it so much, and I found it to be such a key step for me in learning both headstand and forearm stand, that I knew I needed to include it in this book too!

———

You'll need three blocks for this one. As with the previous variation, have your mat at the wall, perpendicular to the wall.

Set up one block, on its highest setting, about an inch away from the wall, with one of the narrow sides facing the wall. Stack the other blocks on top of that one, on their lowest, flat, vertical settings. Make sure the top two blocks are actually touching the wall.

Come onto your forearms and knees and interlace your hands around the bottom block. Stack your shoulders over your elbows and push your forearms into the floor.

Continue to push the floor away with your forearms, and keep your head off the floor, as you tuck your toes, lift your knees, and walk your feet toward the wall until your upper back makes light contact with the blocks.

Lift one leg high and see if you can float the other leg away from the floor to meet it, bringing both heels to the wall. If the back of your head is touching the bottom block, gently press into it. Both this action and the action of gently pressing your upper back into the top blocks can help you balance.

Let your head hang freely with the crown of your head hovering off the mat. If you feel stable, try moving one or both heels off the wall.

Lower down before you feel like you have to, one leg at a time.

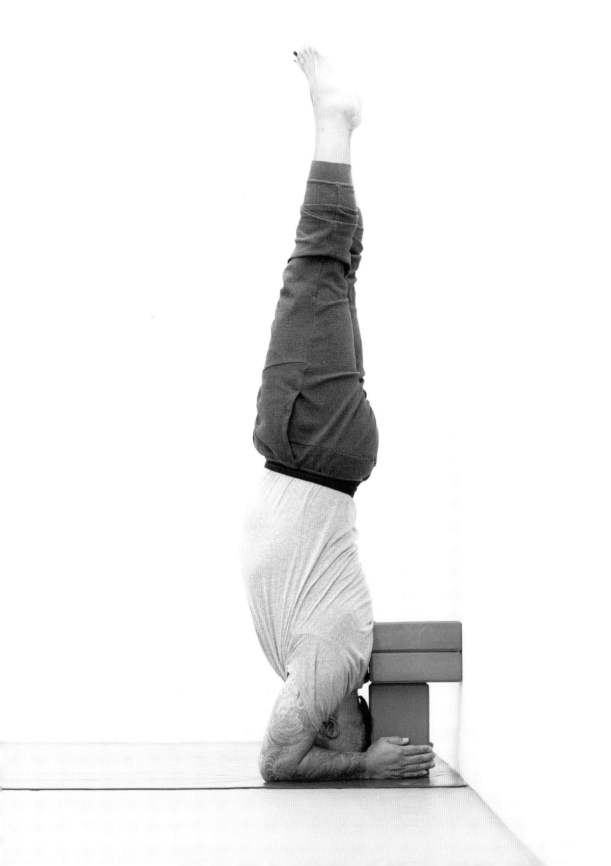

Headstand Prep with Feet on Floor

If you're comfortable with your preferred headless headstand variation, if you've been working with the preps to strengthen and mobilize your shoulders and back, and if bearing weight through your head and neck is not contraindicated for you, you may wish to start moving toward one of the "traditional" forms of sirsasana. The key is to increase the load you're to bear *gradually* in order to set yourself up for success! This prep is a great way to start.

———

Set up as you would for dolphin pose: on forearms and knees with your shoulders stacked over your elbows. Interlace your palms, "cup them" (leave a little space between them), and tuck your bottom pinky in, to avoid crushing your pinky and so that you can press down evenly through the outer edges of your hands, wrists, and forearms, which will take weight out of your head and neck.

Resist your forearms toward each other, reminding yourself to keep up this action so your elbows don't splay. (If they do, that's a sign to come out of the pose for now and go back to the earlier preps to strengthen and mobilize your shoulder girdle.) Continue to press your outer hands, wrists, and forearms *strongly* into the floor, reminding yourself to keep up this too.

Place your crown on the floor so that the back of your head is pressing against the back of your cupped hands (similar to how it was pressing against the bottom block in the "stonehenge" variation on page 132).

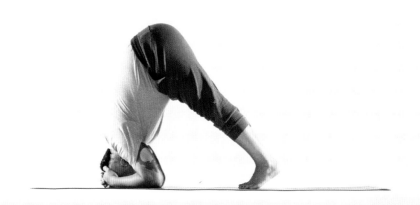

See if you can press your forearms into the floor so much that the crown of your head lifts away from it. Keeping that much engagement, place your crown back down, tuck your toes, lift your knees, and begin to walk your feet toward your head. (If your elbows splay, you've gone too far.) Aim to get your hips *right* up over your shoulders or as close as possible.

Stay for several breaths and then lift your head, walk your feet back, and lower to your knees to release, or try lifting one leg at a time.

Headstand Prep with One Leg Lifted

From the headstand prep above, lift your left leg high in the air, allowing your hip to open if you like, and rising up high onto the ball of your right foot (keep it on the floor for now, though). Stay for a breath or two, continuing to resist your forearms toward each other and to push the floor away with your forearms. Then lower your left foot and repeat on the other side.

To come out, lower your right foot, walk both feet back, and lower your knees to the floor. Lift your head gradually to avoid a head rush, particularly if you're prone to low blood pressure.

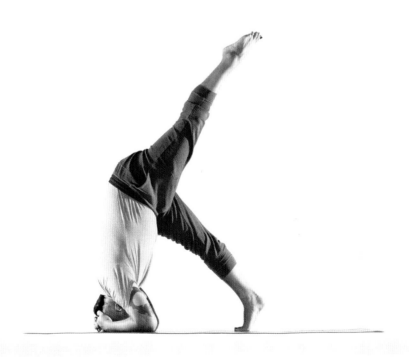

Coming into Sirsasana I One Leg at a Time

Here's a checklist for approaching this one, which you'll come into via the prep we just explored.

When practicing that prep:

- Can you walk your feet forward so that your hips are pretty much over your shoulders?

- Without your elbows splaying?

- While continuing to push the floor away strongly with your outer hands, wrists, and forearms?

- While breathing comfortably?

- And does it feel good?

If you checked all of the above (meaning "yes!"), you're ready to approach liftoff!

From the previous prep, with your left leg reaching high in the air, *continue* to push the floor away until your right toes float off the ground.

You can continue to keep your legs apart or, if you feel balanced, bring your right leg up to meet your left. Hug your legs together and reach up through your inner heels.

Come down before you feel you have to, lowering one leg at a time, and then try again, lifting your right leg first.

Tip: If you're new to headstanding or if a middle-of-the-room headstand doesn't seem appropriate now, try this entrance in front of a wall so you can rest your heels on it. Still be sure to press your forearms into the floor just as much as you would without the wall in order to avoid sinking into your neck and shoulders.

Tuck-Press Entrance

As with one-footed handstand presses (page 76), some folks find a bent-knee approach to coming into headstand works best.

Set up as you did in the previous variation and prep, walking your feet forward until your hips are over your shoulders.

From there, lift your left foot and squeeze your left heel toward your seat.

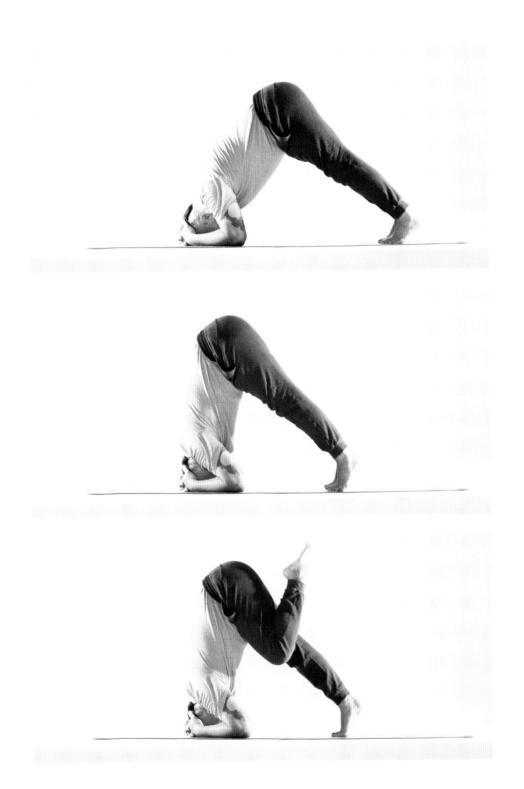

Stay here or see if you can float your right toes off the floor and bend your right knee as well. Initially it might be helpful to keep your knees really close to your torso when you "tuck up," but over time you might be able to lift them away, as Nam is in the photo.

And if you feel balanced and stable, you might even straighten your legs!

Come down with as much control as you can, lowering one straight leg at a time or tucking your legs.

When you're ready, try again, tucking your right leg first.

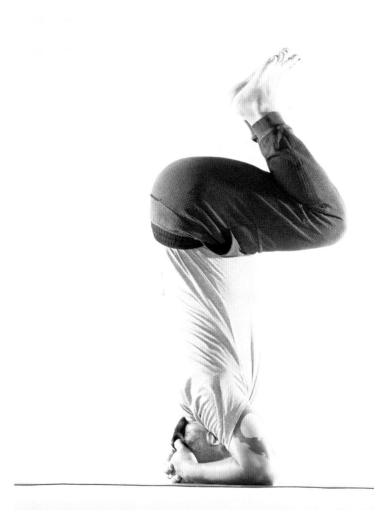

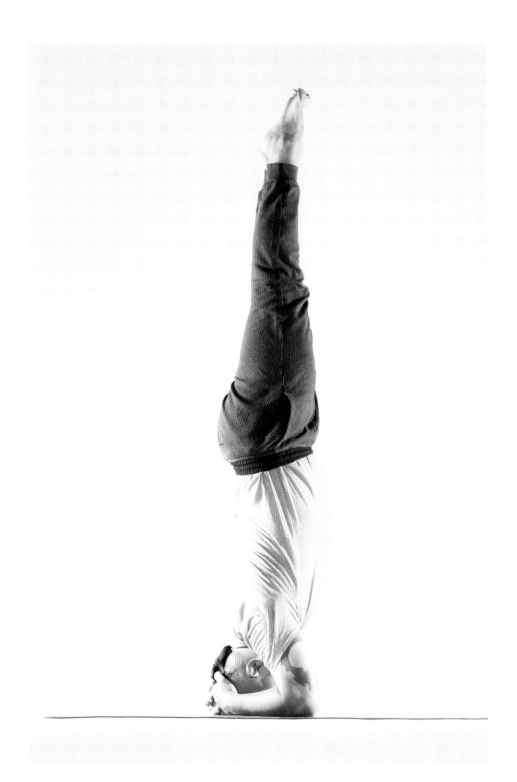

With Feet on the Wall

The wall is my favorite prop, and I love this variation of headstand because I can really press my heels against it, which helps me feel extra-supported, allowing me to remain in the pose longer.

———

Set up with your mat at the wall, perpendicular to it, and come to forearms and knees facing away from the wall, with your toes tucked under and the balls of your feet touching the wall.

Interlace your hands to set up for sirsasana I, just as you did in the previous variations: hands cupped; pinky tucked; outer edges of hands, wrists, and forearms pressing into the floor. Place your crown on the floor so the back of your head presses into your cupped hands.

Resist your forearms in, push the ground away, and lift your knees and hips. Walk your feet up the wall, as you would to come into L pose at the wall (page 44), so that your heels are the same height as your hips.

Really push the ground away and at the same time push your heels into the wall. If this variation is working for you, stay a few breaths. You can also explore lifting one leg at a time in the air if you like.

When you're ready to come down, walk your feet back down the wall.

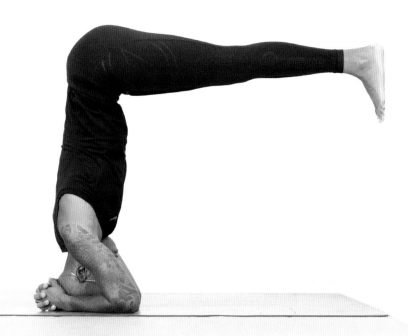

Sirsasana II

I first encountered sirsasana II, also known as a "tripod headstand," in my elementary school gym class. Though it's the first inversion a lot of us learn (thanks in part to school gym classes, I'm sure), it's sometimes considered more "advanced" than sirsasana I because it typically requires more weight-bearing through the head and neck.

On the other end of the "yoga level" spectrum (proving how subjective the idea of "advanced" and "beginner" poses really is), sirsasana II is also used by some folks as a handstand preparation because, thanks to the placement of hands on the floor, it has some similarities in structure and approach to handstand—handstand-press variations in particular. In fact, some people may find it helpful to think of sirsasana II as a press handstand with elbows bent and head on the floor.

As with every pose, there are many ways to approach this one, and you can certainly adapt the entrances for sirsasana I to sirsasana II if you wish. But for the sake of exploring something new, we'll break it down with a wide-leg entrance.

If you'd rather not try it in the middle of the room, you can do this facing a wall, setting up close enough to the wall that you can place your heels on it, but far enough away that you have room to actually get up.

———

Begin in a wide-legged standing forward fold (prasarita padottanasana, like on page 149, but without the hand clasp)—wide enough that you can easily place the top of your head on the mat. Bring your crown to the mat in front of your hands, in a spot where you can see your fingertips, in order to create a triangle. This is your foundation, and these are your points of contact for the inversion: your head and your two hands. Your elbows are bent here, and you want to resist them toward each other (think "chaturanga arms").

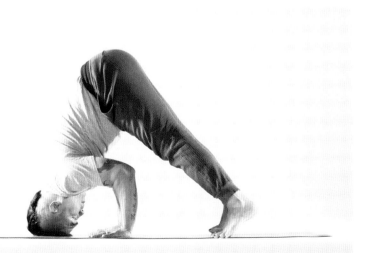

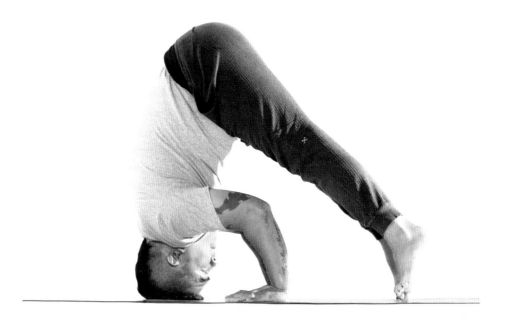

Press your hands into the floor and resist them back toward your feet to take pressure out of your head and neck.

Maintaining those key actions with your hands (pressing down and isometrically resisting back), and continuing to hug your elbows in, start to shift your weight forward as you rise up high on your toes.

Perhaps you can float both feet off the floor in a straddle position (similar to the straddle-press handstand on page 62).

Keep your legs wide as you find your balance. Actively spread your toes, and if you feel steady and ready, draw your legs together. If you do so, squeeze them together and reach up through your heels to continue to lift up out of your foundation.

When you're ready to come down, separate your legs, and lower them back to the floor with just as much control as you used to come up.

Take your time coming out of the pose to avoid a head rush, perhaps lifting your head off the floor and shortening your stance just a bit, enjoying a few breaths in a forward bend, and then transitioning to child's pose for a few breaths before coming upright.

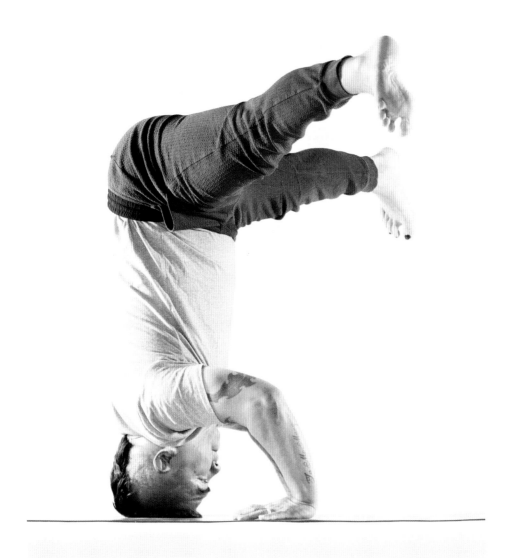

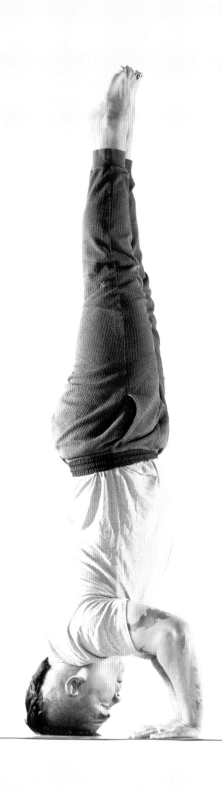

If you'd like a plan for learning to headstand, you can use the one for learning fore-arm stand starting on page 183. Replace the "Forearm Stand Practice" sections of the plan each day with a headstand prep or variation that's appropriate for your current needs and goals. For example, if you're comfortable beginning to bear some weight on your head and neck, you could start with the sirsasana I prep with one leg lifted on page 135. If and when that feels easy, you can explore coming into head-stand with both feet off the floor.

You can also use that time to practice any of the headless headstand variations if you need or want to avoid weight-bearing through your head and neck, or if they just seem like fun!

Feel free to sub any of the drills or stretches in the plan for others (including any of the headstand-specific preps and drills in this chapter, on page 124) with a similar purpose or that better fit your needs.

You can find a blank grid on page 188 in the appendix that you can use to create a custom plan for you or your yoga students.

To learn where and how to include headstand in the context of a complete yoga practice or class, see the sample sequence blueprint on page 195. I prefer to include headstands in the arm balances and arm-balancing inversions sections, but others like to include them close to the end of practice, before savasana.

Headstand (Sirsasana)

Shoulderstand (Salamba Sarvangasana)
+ Plow Pose (Halasana)

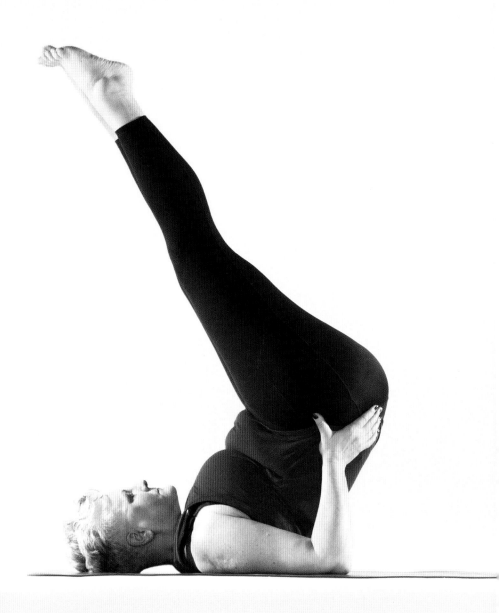

My first yoga memory is related to shoulder-stand and plow. My mom used to do both at the end of her regular workout routine in our living room, and as a toddler, I'd stand around waiting with bated breath for her to transition into plow so that I could jump on her back. (Sorry about that, Mom. Glad your spine is okay!)

Though my mom would often incorporate various asanas into her workout and stretching routines, I didn't realize those poses were "yoga" until one of my favorite cartoons (an anime called *Adventures of the Little Koala*, which was broadcast on Nickelodeon in the '80s and '90s) told me so. This was great news, because I loved doing those poses myself as I watched TV or played in the grass. Who knew little me could do yoga?

Back then, those inversions were often presented in media as quintessential depictions of yoga, but they've fallen out of favor in recent years. As with headstand, they've gained a bit of a negative reputation in the yoga world (see "Why Headstand Gets a Bad Rap" on page 123). These days, flashier inversions and arm balances such as scorpion pose (a handstand or fore-arm stand that incorporates a backbend and bending your knees to bring your toes toward your head) are more likely to be used to depict "yoga" in probiotic ads and on cereal boxes.

But I think there's still value we can gain from shoulderstand and plow. That doesn't mean that they're for everyone, but a lot of folks (including my husband, Kyle, who is demonstrating many of the variations you'll find in this chapter) really love these poses. And understandably, it can be kind of disheart-ening to constantly hear that a pose that feels great for you is "injurious," "outdated," or "bad."

Not every pose is for everyone, but if you enjoy plow and shoulderstand and your tissues have adapted to the load that these poses require you to bear, there's no reason to remove them from your practice, particularly if you're using props (which I recommend for these poses for most people, most of the time).

And if you'd like to learn them but aren't sure where to begin or how to make them work for your body, good news! That's what this chapter is all about: showing a variety of approaches and options and sharing tips and tricks that can help you make them work for *you*.

BENEFITS

Similar to headstand being nicknamed the "king of asanas," shoulderstand is often called "the queen." (So what does that make plow? The court jester? A duke of some sort? I have questions.) And just like headstand, shoulderstand is often said to offer a whole host of benefits, some more believable than others. Like I actually just read an online article that says shoulderstand can aid in weight loss and that it "reduces the extra flap present around the stomach." Okay, first, weight loss is *not* a universal "benefit." It's not something everyone is interested in, nor is it healthy for everyone. Can we stop with that already? Ditto for the "stomach flap." What year is this again? Can we just quit with the body shaming and bad science? I'm stepping off my soapbox now, but feel free to google "benefits of shoulderstand" if you'd like to be both horrified and/or get a good laugh. My favorite was "promotes hair growth." I had to stop when I got to "cure diabetes." *No. It will not do that*.

But folks can experience *actual* benefits from practicing shoulderstand and plow and their variations, which include increased circulation of blood and lymph. Some people also say that it has helped them to facilitate better breathing and increase their lung capacity, alleviate digestive discomfort (as someone with IBS, I can personally attest to this; your mileage may vary), and cultivate a general sense of well-being.

Most of all, when I ask people why they like these poses, they respond with a big smile and say, "Because they *feel* good!" And as far as I'm concerned, that's the best reason of all to practice them, and the same reason why I practiced them all those years ago in my living room and on my front lawn.

GENERAL CONTRAINDICATIONS

As always, talk to your medical provider if you have any questions about poses or movements that may be contraindicated for you. In general, the "traditional" forms of these poses are considered contraindicated for untreated high blood pressure, glaucoma or any condition where you need to avoid increased eye pressure, and neck injuries.

A note about menstruation and pregnancy: "Traditionally" menstruation is considered a contraindication, but if you've read the "Myths about Inversions" section on page 10, you already know my thoughts on that one. Pregnancy is also a still-oft-repeated contraindication, and while I wouldn't recommend trying shoulderstand or plow for the first time if you're currently pregnant, if you've been practicing them regularly and your health-care provider has given you the okay, there's no reason why you can't continue to do them as long as they're comfortable for you.

Standing Wide-Legged Forward Fold with Hand Clasp or Strap (Prasarita Padottanasana C)

Purpose: To stretch your chest, shoulders, and hamstrings in a standing pose that resembles the shape of plow. This forward bend is also a mild inversion in its own right.

In Practice: Take a wide stance with your knees and toes pointing in the same direction. Interlace your hands behind your back, bringing your palms as close together as you comfortably can. You can also hold a yoga strap, belt, pet leash, or towel between your hands if that feels better. Keep a little bend in your elbows, which can help broaden your chest. Inhale here, and exhale, fold forward.

Stay for five to ten breaths before rising back up to standing.

Tip: For a more restorative variation (which can also be a great alternative to plow), support your head with props such as blocks, blankets, or bolsters.

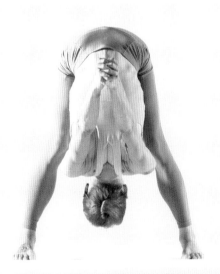

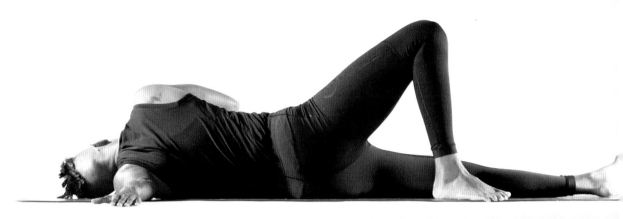

Swimmer's Stretch

Purpose: This is called "swimmers stretch" because it's often used by swimmers after practice to relieve tight chest and shoulder muscles, increase range of motion, and prevent "swimmer's shoulder." It's useful for us land dwellers too and an excellent way to stretch and mobilize those areas for shoulderstand and plow.

In Practice: Lie face down on your belly. Place your right hand under your shoulder, as you would for cobra pose, and reach your left arm out to a T shape—at or slightly above shoulder height—palm facing down. Inhale here, and as you exhale, begin to roll onto your left side, first stacking your right leg over your left. Rest the left side of your head on the mat, a block, or in any position that feels comfortable, and aim to stack your left shoulder over your right in order to stretch your chest and the fronts of your shoulders.

If this feels like a good stretch, stay here. To intensify the stretch, bend your right knee and bring the ball of your right foot, perhaps even the entire sole of your right foot, to the ground behind your left leg, as Shanté is demonstrating in the photo.

Remain in the pose for five to ten breaths, then roll back onto your belly and change sides.

Restorative Fish Pose (*Matsyasana*)

Purpose: In many yoga sequences, including those in the Ashtanga yoga series, fish pose is done as a counter pose *after* shoulderstand and plow. But I think this restorative version is a great preparation for those inversions as well! That's because it's a gentle, passive way to release your chest and shoulders, which can make those poses easier to get into and stay in. And because you're supported by props, you can lie back and enjoy this pose for longer than your typical active backbend. This is an especially nice option for folks like me who find backbends to be challenging in general!

In Practice: Set up two blocks on your mat—the first on its highest height right at the back edge of your mat, and the second at its medium height about eighteen inches or so from the back edge of your mat. This is just a starting point; you may need to adjust your blocks as you go. Your blocks can either be horizontal or vertical (i.e., on the wide or narrow setting) depending on your block type and what feels best for your body.

Sit in front of your block setup on your mat with your knees bent and feet on the floor, then lie back over the blocks so that your shoulder blades are supported by the second block (I like to line up the bottom tips of my shoulder blades with the bottom edge of the block as a reference point) and the back of your skull is supported by the first block. Adjust the height and position of the blocks as needed for optimum comfort. You can keep your arms alongside you, as Sarah is in the photo, or bring them into any position you like. Reaching your arms overhead (perhaps clasping opposite elbows) can intensify the stretch if desired.

Keep your knees bent, stretch them out long, or bring them into a butterfly position—whatever feels good! Stay for a minute or two and come out slowly in a manner that's comfortable for you, perhaps using your hands to gently press up to seated (lead with your chest so your head comes up last) or mindfully rolling onto a side and pressing to an upright seat from there.

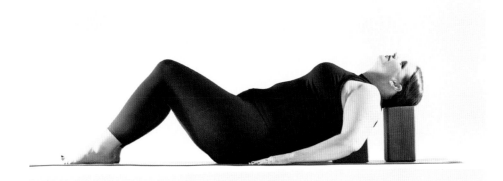

Seated Forward Fold (*Paschimottanasana*)

Purpose: Paschimottanasana is essentially plow pose upside down. (Or should that be "right side up"? The point is, it's a seated forward fold that resembles the shape of plow.) It will stretch your hamstrings and back muscles in preparation for plow.

In Practice: Sit tall on your mat with your legs out in front of you, your feet flexed, and your arms alongside you. Begin with a long, neutral spine. If your lower back rounds (which it will for most of us), sit on the edge of a folded blanket or two in order to maintain the natural inward curve of your lower back. Starting this way will make it easier to fold forward. You might also find it helpful to bend your knees a little bit. (This is an especially helpful tip if your lower back rounds when sitting upright and you don't have any props on hand.)

Inhale, try to lengthen your spine even more, and on an exhale, keep your spine long as you hinge forward from your hip creases, walking your hands forward toward your feet. At some point your spine will round and no longer be in its neutral position, and even as it does, still prioritize a *long* spine so you don't (for example) have way more rounding in your upper back than your lower back—allow *all* of your spinal muscles to enjoy the stretch! As you release in the fold, you can rest your hands on the ground, or hold your feet and ankles, or use a strap around your feet if you have one.

With every inhale, see if you can lengthen the front of your torso a little more, and with every exhale, see if you can fold a bit deeper.

Stay for five to ten breaths, then rise back up with a long spine on an inhale.

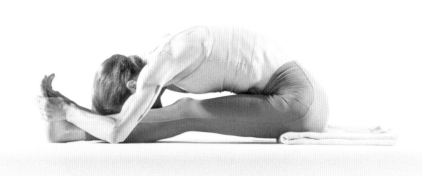

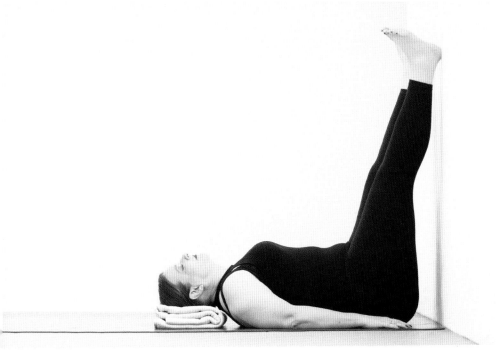

Legs-Up-the-Wall Pose Variations

These variations share many benefits with shoulderstand, but they can be better options for folks with a history of neck or shoulder injuries. Many of these variations also keep the head at the same level as the heart, so if, like Sarah, inverting in general is contraindicated for you, you may still be able to reap the rewards of shoulderstand. Legs-up-the-wall pose in particular is *great* for relieving swelling in your feet and ankles.

And a pretty cool bonus: once, after an especially exhausting day, I accidentally fell asleep in legs-up-the-wall pose (it really can be *that* relaxing), and now I can technically say that I held an inversion for over an hour!

Start by sitting with your right hip against a wall, as close to it as possible. Then turn to the right, roll onto your back, and bring your legs up the wall. Your legs can be slightly bent if you like, and they can be neutral or turned out—whatever is most relaxing for you.

If the back of your neck feels compressed, or if you'd just like the extra comfort, slide a folded blanket (or a pillow) under your head. Your hips don't have to touch the wall completely, but feel free to scoot your buttocks closer toward it if you'd like.

Keep your arms alongside your body or place them in any position that feels good. Assuming you don't fall asleep like I did, stay for three to five minutes. When you're ready to come out, bend your knees, place your feet on the wall, and roll onto one side. Stay there for a breath or two before pressing up to seated.

If you'd like to turn this into just a *little* more of an inversion, bringing your heart just slightly above your head, you can elevate your hips with a bolster or folded blanket(s), like Kyle. And to get a little more chest and shoulder opening, bring your arms into the goalpost position he's demonstrating in the photo or reach them straight overhead.

The version Shanté is doing here, with a strap snuggly around her shins, is my favorite because with the strap keeping my legs in place, I don't have to exert any effort at all to prevent them from splaying. I can just lie back, chill out, and enjoy. (Place the strap around your legs before bringing them up the wall.)

Another option for making this pose extra relaxing is to place a sandbag on the soles of your feet like Sarah. If you don't have a sandbag, try a bag of rice, a heavy folded blanket, or even some bean bags. (If you're from the Midwest like me, you might have some lying around from your last game of cornhole!) To come into this one, have the sandbag within reach, but bring your legs up the wall first. Then bend your knees, sliding your heels down the wall enough so that you can grab your sandbag, place it over the soles of your feet, then slide your legs back up. When you're ready to come out, bend your knees again, slide your heels back down, and remove the sandbag before rolling onto your side to sit up.

Or if you happen to have a willing pal nearby, you can ask them to place and remove the sandbag for you.

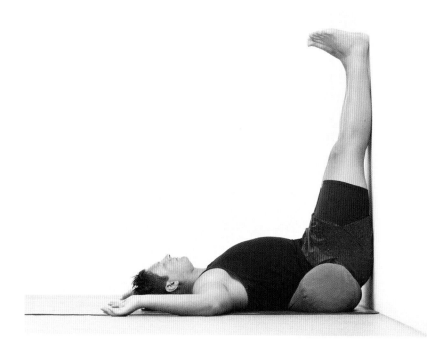

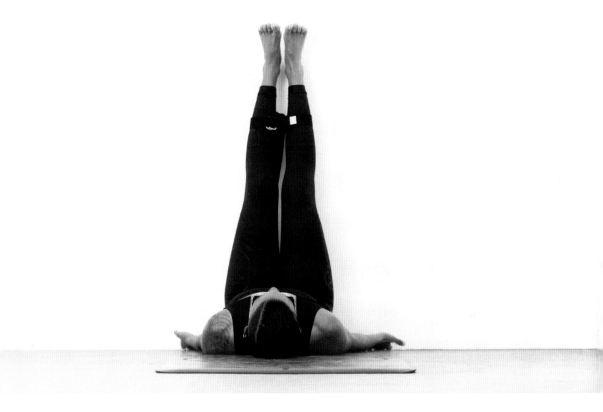

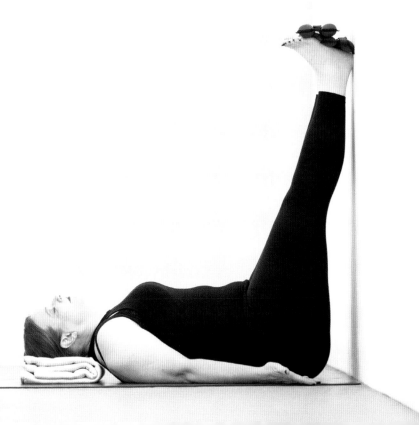

Also referred to as "half shoulderstand," viparita karani variations are a great way to approach shoulderstand, and they're a fabulous alternative for anyone who wants to explore a position more inverted than what legs-up-the-wall pose offers without bearing a lot of weight through the shoulders and neck. It also happens to be my favorite version of shoulderstand.

With a Block

Practicing with a block is a little more "active" than legs up the wall but still gives you some extra support so you can stay in the pose longer. It's also nice for folks who have sore wrists and don't want to support their pelvis with their hands.

To try it, lie on your back with your knees bent, feet flat on the floor and a block within reach. Make sure there's a little bit of space between the back of your neck and the floor. Lift your hips away from the floor, as you would for bridge pose, and place the block, at any height you like, under your pelvis. The exact placement depends on what feels most supportive to you, but avoid placing the block right under your lower back, which tends to get uncomfortable for a lot of folks after they've been in the pose for a while. Let the weight of your pelvis settle into the block, adjusting its position or height as needed. Once the block is stable in place, in a position that feels good for you, stretch your legs up to the sky, one at a time. Keep your palms alongside you or bring your hands to any position that's comfortable. For more chest and shoulder opening, you can bring your arms to a cactus position or straighten them overhead, palms up.

Stay for five to ten breaths, or a little longer if you'd like, then return your arms alongside you if you moved them, lift your hips to remove the block, and release your pelvis back to the floor.

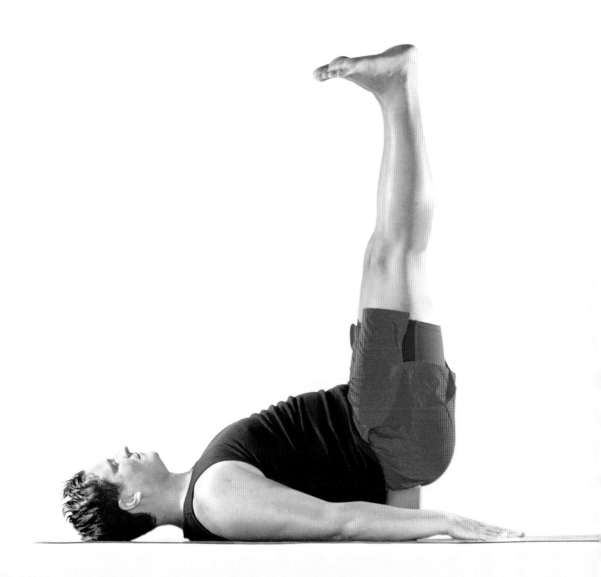

Without a Block

As with the previous version, set up in bridge pose on your mat, lifting your hips off the floor. Walk your shoulder blades toward each other to broaden your chest and bring your hands to the back of your pelvis, so you're holding it as Peggy is. Your hands are doing in this version what the block was doing in the previous version. Before you lift your legs, walk your shoulder blades closer in so that your elbows are shoulder-width apart or closer. If they are, that's your signal that it's okay to lift your legs. Lift one leg at a time, supporting your pelvis with your hands. Remember: you're not going all the way up into a shoulderstand here, with your legs pointing straight up. (I don't typically recommend doing that without props in place to help you maintain the curve of your neck.) Your legs should be at more of an angle, as Peggy's are. Note that the farther away from your face your legs go, the more pressure this will be on your wrists; adjust the position of your hands and the angle of your legs as needed (perhaps moving them farther from your face) to find the position most comfortable for you. Keep your upper body as is, though, to avoid weight-bearing through your shoulders and neck.

Stay for about five to ten breaths before returning your feet to the floor, one at a time, releasing your hands, and lowering your pelvis to the floor.

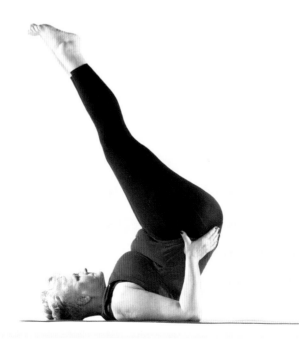

With a Block and a Strap

Instead of intensifying inverted action pose by removing props, you can make it even *more* restorative by using a strap to keep your legs in place, allowing you to let go of some effort.

———

Start by making a big loop with your strap. As with any prop-enhanced variation, you may need to experiment to figure out what's just right for you, so it could take a few tries to find the right-size loop. If one strap doesn't cut it (which is likely if you're pretty tall; you may also benefit from a longer strap if you have a wider torso, tighter legs or hips, or a tighter lower back), you can connect two straps together to make a longer loop.

Slip the strap around your torso, just below your armpits, with the buckle in a place that will be in reach (near the front of your body, close to your hand) so that you can adjust the strap to make it tauter or looser as needed. Then lie down on your back to set up for bridge pose with a block in reach.

Lift your hips to place the block under your pelvis to support it. Lift one foot off the floor, knee bent, and loop the bottom of the strap over the arch. Then do the same with the other foot. If you still feel well supported by the block, and if your

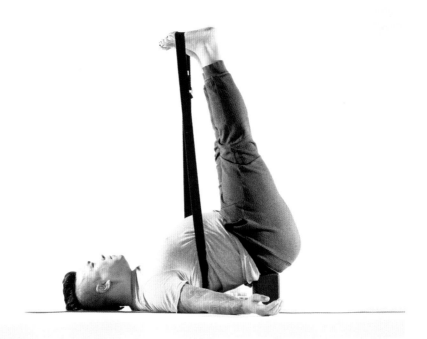

strap is long enough, start to straighten your legs up toward the sky, flexing your feet and pushing them into the strap. (If not, adjust your strap if you're able, or lower down and adjust your props, then try again.)

Stay for five to ten breaths or more. To come down, bend your knees and slide the strap off your feet, releasing them to the floor one at a time. Lift your pelvis to remove the block, then lower it to the floor. Roll onto a side, press up to seated, and then remove yourself from the strap.

With Strap around Chest

Peggy is demonstrating this tried-and-true hack in inverted action pose, but you can use it to make any shoulderstand variation more comfortable if you have a larger chest. (The effects of gravity can make it difficult for some folks to breathe in this pose, and the strap provides a space-making solution.)

Before you come into the pose, loop a strap around the top of your chest and under your armpits, cinching it firmly in place. Adjust if and as needed and then lie back and breathe freely in the inversion!

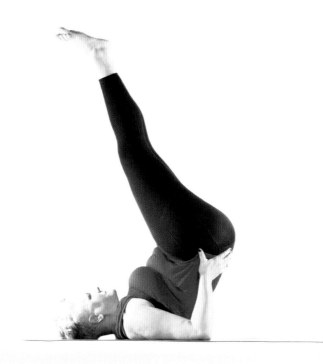

With a Bolster and Chair

I think of myself as a prop minimalist. I adore yoga props for both progressing and regressing poses as I need to, but I get overwhelmed by too many. So when my pal Nam mentioned a variation of viparita karani that involved a chair, blankets, *and* a bolster, I was skeptical. But once he showed it to me and I tried it for myself, I was sold and knew I had to share it with you in this book. (Thanks, Nam!)

———

To try it yourself, open up a folding chair and place it on your mat as pictured, upside down so that the legs are in the air and pointing away from you, toward the front edge of the mat, and the chairback and seat are making an inverted V shape on the floor.

Drape one blanket over the bar between the two highest chair legs. For a little added luxury, place a thinly folded blanket on the mat right behind the chair, so that when you're in the pose, your head, neck, and shoulders will be off the blanket as pictured.

Finally, place a bolster vertically over the chairback.

From there, sit on the bolster, swing your legs up over the bar with the draped blanket, then use your hands to guide you as you slowly lower onto your back.

You could extend your arms out into a T shape, bend them into a cactus shape like Nam, or reach them up overhead.

If you're anything like me, you'll want to stay in this one a *long* time. Three to five minutes feels great, but enjoy it for longer if you like.

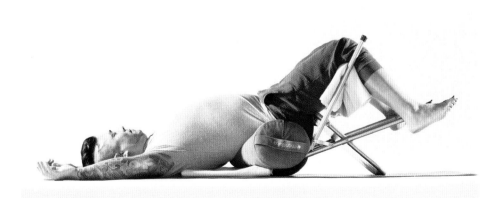

SHOULDERSTAND VARIATIONS

The Sanskrit name for the pose we usually call shoulderstand is salamba sarvangasana, which literally translates to "supported whole-body pose." You could take that to mean that your whole body is held supported over your shoulders, which it is in the most commonly depicted version, but I like to think of the "supported" part of the moniker as a reminder that most of us will really benefit from the support of props in this pose. In these variations, I recommend using props to help you maintain the curve of your neck, which in general makes the pose more sustainable and more comfortable. There are many different ways to do this (you might already have a favorite), and the exact setup and number of blankets, mats, or other props you use will depend on your unique structure—there is no "one size fits all."

As you figure out the right support, here are some general guidelines and landmarks to keep in mind:

- In shoulderstand (and plow), you want your head and neck *off* the props and on your mat in order to maintain your cervical (neck) curve.

- Your shoulders, however, will be *on* the props.

- You'll naturally scoot back a little (toward the back of your mat, in the direction the crown of your head is pointing) getting into shoulderstand, so set up just a little bit forward of where you'll ultimately want to be. If you're an anatomy geek who likes to get super specific, you might find this tip that Karina, one of my very first yoga teachers, mentioned on page 121, shared with me helpful: ultimately aim to have your C7 vertebra (that's the big one right at the base of your neck) *on* the props and the rest of your cervical vertebrae (all those other smaller neck bones) *off* the props, maintaining your cervical curve (the natural curve of your neck).

- Use as many well-folded, evenly stacked blankets as you need to preserve your cervical curve. Most folks need more than one. I usually recommend two to start.

- Fold your yoga mat over your blanket(s) as Nam is in the photos that follow, which adds traction and prevents you from slipping. (You will notice that Nam is using an extra folded yoga mat in lieu of a second blanket, which creates just the right prop height for him, but may or may not be the case for you. The important thing is that you maintain the curve of your neck, not the number of blankets you do or don't use.)

Note: As I alluded to on page 147, shoulderstand is one of the more controversial asanas—perhaps even the most controversial—and there are many different approaches to it and schools of thought about it. The recommendations here are ones that I have found helpful for myself and the students I work with, but there are certainly many very good yoga teachers who would disagree with my approach completely. And that's okay. Remember that all bodies are different, and we as humans are constantly learning new things about how our bodies work, how they differ from one another, and how they get strong and heal. If something doesn't work for you or resonate with you, or if you just don't feel confident or convinced about a particular variation or tip, skip it.

Alright. That's it with the housekeeping. If you're still with me, let's break down how to get into shoulderstand and explore some variations.

With Blankets and a Mat

Fold two blankets (add more if needed) into even rectangles and stack them so that the folds line up evenly and the folded "clean" edges of the blankets are closer to the back of your mat (this is the part that will be supporting your shoulders).

Place a folded sticky mat on top of the blankets or drape the bottom of your practice mat over them, like Nam is, for traction. Some people prefer to drape the mat only over the first two-thirds of the blanket stack, while others like to cover it completely.

Lie back over the blankets so your shoulders are supported by them and your head is on the floor, with your shoulders just a little farther forward (toward the front of the mat, in the direction your feet are pointing) than they will be when you come up.

Bend your knees and place your feet on the floor as you would for bridge pose, and rest your arms alongside you.

My preference is to come into bridge pose first, lifting my hips, and then to transition as I would to come into inverted action pose (page 156), walking my shoulder blades toward each other, holding my pelvis with my hands, and then bringing my shoulder blades in even closer so that my elbows are shoulder-width or closer (a prerequisite for coming up).

From there, I'll lift one foot then the other to come into viparita karani first. Then if I'm still feeling good, I'll start to walk my hands "down" my back (closer to my shoulders) until my legs are as vertical as they comfortably can be and I'm still maintaining the curve of my neck and breathing comfortably.

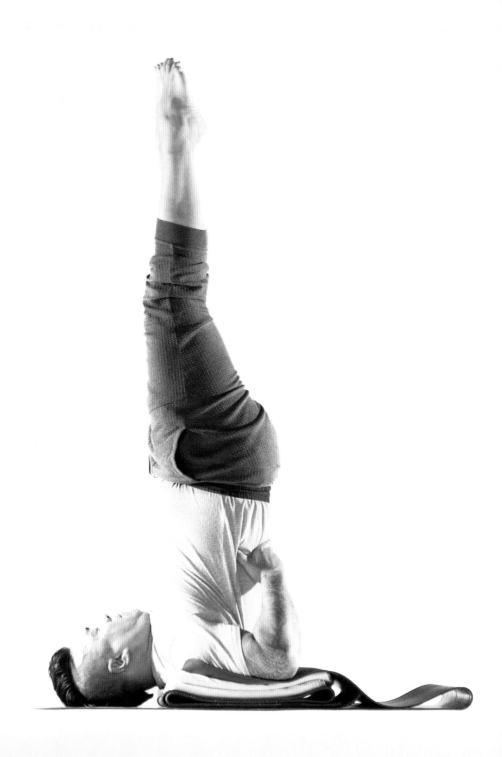

In lieu of the bridge setup, which takes a good amount of strength and control (and occasionally a little help from a favorite yoga teacher to get into), some people prefer the following:

Start lying back over the blankets with arms alongside you, knees bent and feet on the floor like the bridge setup, but instead of lifting your hips to come into bridge, push your hands and feet into the floor and use a bit of momentum to lift your feet, draw your thighs toward your torso, curl your pelvis up, and rock back into the pose with control, catching hold of your pelvis and walking your hands down your spine in the process.

If you prefer this option, remember to not use so much momentum that you slide off your props or lose control but just enough to get up there.

Once you're in the pose, check in: Are your shoulders (and perhaps that C7 vertebra) still on the props? Is your head off the props? Is there space between the back of your neck and the mat? Are you comfortable? Can you breathe? If not, come down, adjust as needed, and try again.

If and when you feel good in the pose, stay for five to ten breaths to start, or longer if you'd like, but only as long as you can maintain your ideal alignment.

To come out, either walk your hands closer to your pelvis (the reverse of how you entered if you came in from bridge) and then lower one foot at a time to return to bridge, releasing your hands and lowering your pelvis. Or bend your knees and roll down slowly, with as much control as you can muster.

And when you're done, that restorative fish pose on page 151 makes a great follow-up.

At the Wall

This is a wonderful variation if you want to approach shoulderstand with a little extra support and control.

————

Bring the short edge of your mat against a wall and place your folded blanket(s) near the opposite end. Lie down over them so that your upper back is on them and your head is not. The tops of your shoulders will be a little more forward of the blanket edges than where they'll end up, because you'll shift back a bit coming into the pose.

Bend your knees and place the bottoms of your feet on the wall. Press your feet into the wall as you lift your pelvis and bring your shoulder blades in closer to each other. Bring your hands to your pelvis, as in viparita karani (page 158). At this point, your weight is still supported by your upper back and not over your shoulders. Keep pressing into the wall and draw your shoulder blades in more so that your elbows are shoulder-width or closer.

You can remain in a wall-enhanced viparita karani or walk your hands "down" your back, coming into a more vertical position, bringing more weight over your shoulders and adjusting your feet as needed. Be sure that there's still space between your neck and the floor.

Stay here for five to ten breaths or longer if you feel good. If you're feeling stable, you can experiment with lifting one leg or both away from the wall.

When you're ready to come out, return your feet to the wall if needed and exit with control, adjusting your feet as needed as you bring your hands back to the floor and slowly lower your hips to the floor.

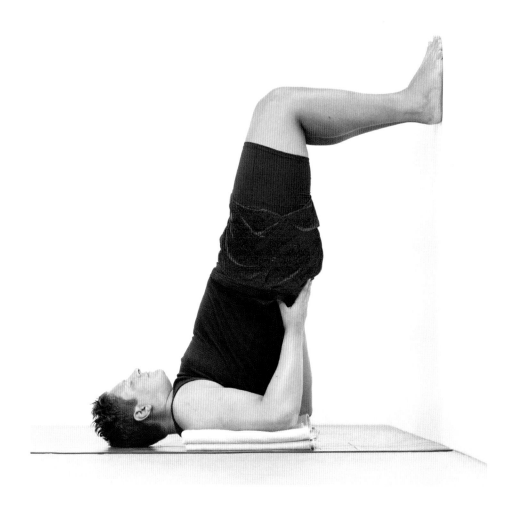

With a Chair

If you've been practicing inverted action pose and think you might be ready to move toward a traditional shoulderstand, this variation is a great stepping-stone because it allows you to increase the load gradually, bringing more weight over your shoulders but not *as* much as the chairless version since your pelvis is supported by the chair seat.

This variation is also a perfect example of how not every version of a pose works for every body. Here's a behind-the-scenes tidbit: I was planning to model this one myself, but after much trial and error, it just wasn't happening. My proportions simply wouldn't allow me to comfortably grab hold of the chair while maintaining my comfortable neck and shoulder alignment, and resting my pelvis on the chair just didn't feel good. Then Kyle kindly agreed to model in my stead. He got into the pose effortlessly and said it felt great! He probably could have stayed there all day.

If this variation (or any variation of any pose) doesn't work for you, don't sweat it. We're all different, and that's why there are so many options out there.

But if you suspect that, like Kyle, this shoulderstand might be one you'll really savor, here's how to do it:

———

Place a yoga chair or folding chair on your mat so that all four legs are on it. A lot of people like to place a folded blanket on the chair seat for added padding. (Kyle apparently has a pelvis of steel and chose to go without one.)

Place your folded blanket/mat setup for shoulderstand on the floor in front of the chair legs to support the curve of your neck in the pose. (As always, adjusting the exact position of your props can take trial and error.)

Then sit on the chair backward, with your legs wide, as though you were the "cool substitute teacher" trying to "rap with the kids." (If you've ever seen an '80s movie where teens are trying to save the rec center, you know exactly what I'm talking about.)

Grasp the sides of the chairback and swing your legs over the upper rim of the backrest, knees bent, similar to how your legs drape in the chair-supported viparita karani on page 161, and begin to slowly lower your back toward the floor. Your legs will automatically start to straighten as you lower, but keep your lower legs resting on the chair's backrest for now. As you approach the floor, bring one hand at a time to grasp the back legs of the chair. (If you have broad shoulders like Kyle, holding on to the outside of the chair legs may feel best; others may prefer to reach between the legs to grab hold.)

Once your shoulders come to the blanket(s) with your head on the mat, your cervical curve maintained, if you feel stable with your pelvis supported on the chair

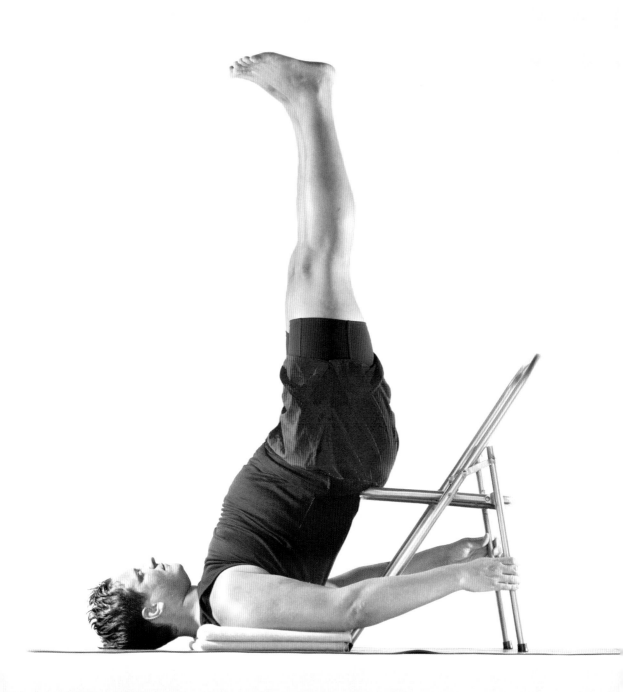

seat, bend one knee at a time toward your chest, then straighten one leg at a time up toward the sky.

And if it feels great, enjoy! Stay for five to ten breaths or longer if you like.

To exit, bend one knee at a time and return your feet to the rim of the backrest. Straighten your legs so you're back where you were before you drew your knees in toward you.

Then, with control, using your hands to help as needed, perhaps bringing them to the front chair legs as you transition, slink your whole back down to the floor and your pelvis onto the blankets that were once supporting your shoulders. Let your lower legs rest on the chair seat with your knees bent. If you're familiar with "legs-over-the-chair pose," that's where you'll end up. Rest your hands wherever is comfortable, alongside you, on your belly.

Enjoy a few breaths here, then roll onto one side, sliding off the blankets and chair with control. Take yet a few more breaths on your side, then press up to seated.

PLOW VARIATIONS

With Blankets and a Mat

In many yoga practices, including the Ashtanga yoga series and many of the styles influenced by Ashtanga, plow pose follows shoulderstand directly.

———

To enter plow from shoulderstand, use the same blanket/mat setup as described on page 163.

From shoulderstand, lower one leg at a time to or toward the floor behind you. This is usually done with ankles flexed and toes tucked, though sometimes I like to point my toes and rest the tops of my feet on the floor.

You can keep your hands supporting your pelvis, place your hands on the floor with palms down, clasp your hands, or reach back toward your feet like Nam.

Stay for five to ten breaths.

Note: Often, such as in Ashtanga and related styles, there are a few other poses you would do before lowering down, but for simplicity's sake we'll exit from here, which is generally my preference when practicing and teaching plow. However, if you'd like to explore these other options, I recommend checking out one of the many wonderful Ashtanga books from Kino MacGregor.

To release, you could come back into shoulderstand and come out in your preferred manner.

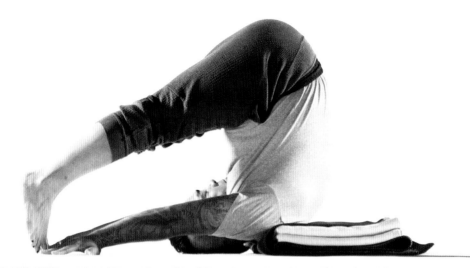

Another option is to simply bring your hands to the floor alongside you, palms down, if they're not already there, and roll down with control.

You can also come right into plow without making a stopover in shoulderstand. You'll still use the same prop setup to support your shoulders (head on the mat, cervical curve intact).

To come straight into plow, lie over your props as if you were going into shoulderstand: just slightly more forward than you'll want to end up in the pose, shoulders on the blankets, head off. Press your hands and feet into the floor and on an exhale, use a tiny bit of momentum to curl your pelvis up, roll back, and bring your feet overhead.

Variation: If you don't have props available and feel comfortable practicing viparita karani unsupported (page 158), you can do a "viparita karani version" of plow where your weight is supported by your upper back instead of over your shoulders. Your hips won't be right over your shoulders in this version and your feet might not touch the floor, so if you like, you can rest them on your couch, your bed, a chair, a wall—whatever's nearby and works.

In the following photos, Kyle is demonstrating the chair and the wall versions while incorporating a couple of different blanket setups, which still may be ideal or necessary for some folks in order to maintain their cervical curve.

These are also great "intermediate" steps for approaching a traditional hips-over-shoulders plow pose because they increase the load gradually. Notice how Kyle's hips are not right up over his shoulders here, so he's not balancing as much weight over them as he would be if he were doing a more "stacked" version like Nam in the photo above.

With a Chair

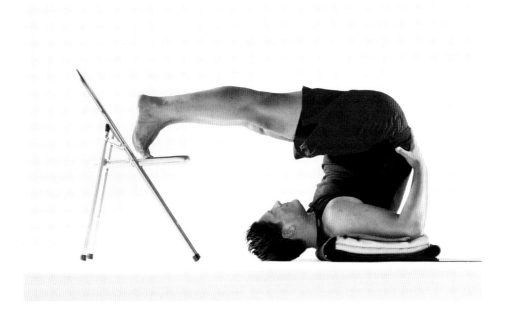

At a Wall

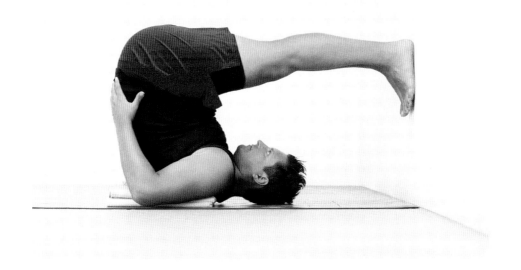

INCORPORATING SHOULDERSTAND, PLOW, AND VARIATIONS IN PRACTICE

Because there are so many variables at hand when it comes to finding a shoulder-stand or plow variation to fit your needs and goals, instead of offering a one-month plan for this section, I encourage you to incorporate any of the preps and variations into your practice as it makes sense for you, adding or subtracting them as your practice grows and changes. And if you're a teacher, to use any of these options to support students if and as appropriate. Of course, change, adapt, and innovate as you like!

For ideas and suggestions on how to do so, you can look at the sample blueprint in appendix 2 on page 195. You can also use the practice grid on page 188 to create your own plan, or a plan for students and clients if you'd like, adding in the preps and poses that make sense for you.

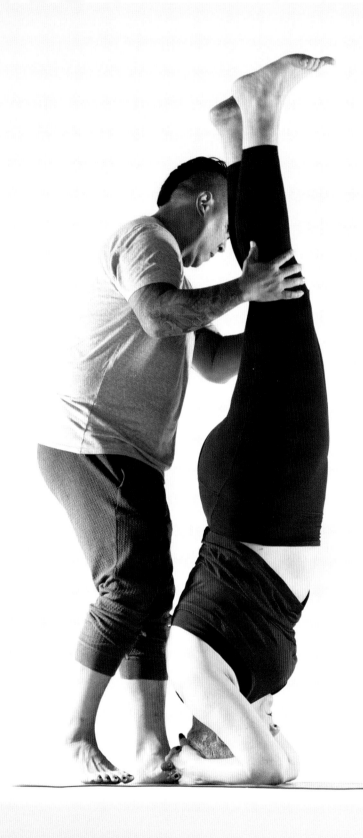

Acknowledgments

This book is possible thanks to the kindness, support, and generosity of more folks than I can mention here, but in particular I want to acknowledge the following people:

Sarah Stanton, for giving me the idea for this book.

My editor, Beth Frankl, for her encouragement and guidance, and all of the folks at Shambhala Publications: truly, you are the best!

My mom, Laura Heagberg, for always reminding me that the best reason to practice inversions is because they feel good. And more importantly, for always having my back, even when I was jumping on hers in plow pose all those years ago.

To Linda Sparrowe, for supporting me throughout my editorial career and believing in me always, even when it was hard to believe in myself.

To my photographer, Annie: you are one of my favorite collaborators and a friend for life.

To all of the models in this book: Shanté, for somehow knowing just how I need to be inspired. Peggy, I'm so glad to know you and to have another sushi buddy! Sarah, you're not only my family but my friend; I've known you most of my life and I've never stopped wanting to be just like you. Nam, you are an incredible friend and you inspired so much in this book—I owe you one again. And to Kyle, who turns my world upside down in all the best ways. I love you. Ham.

Special thanks to Athleta and Superfit Hero for providing wardrobe for this book and offering inclusive sizing options.

Appendix 1
Practice Grids

TAKING YOUR HANDSTAND OFF THE WALL: DAY 1

WARM-UP				
Spend a few breaths moving in downward-facing dog (walking in place, etc.) + follow with a few wrist stretches. (These can be the same wrist stretches below in the mobility/stretch portion, or anything else you like!)				
DRILLS, HIIT-STYLE 4 sets total, alternating exercises A through D (like a circuit). Alternate 30 seconds of work, 10 seconds of rest.				
	Purpose	Exercise	Sets	Reps or duration	Rest
A	Upper-body strength/core + spinal stability	Plank walks (page 98)	4	30 seconds	10 seconds
B	Endurance, momentum, hip mobility	Yoga burpees (page 30)	4	30 seconds	10 seconds
C	Core strength; give your wrists a break!	Hollow hold (page 35)	4	30 seconds	10 seconds
D	Upper-body strength, core strength, endurance, shifting weight into fingertips	Mountain climbers (page 29)	4	30 seconds	10 seconds

MOBILITY + FLEXIBILITY WORK

	Purpose	Exercise	Sets	Reps or duration	Rest
1	Wrist stretches	Choose 1–2 from the tips on page 92	1	1–2 minutes each/each side	None
2	Hip flexibility/mobility	Pigeon (page 36) or firelog pose (page 36)	1	2–3 minutes each side	None
3	Hip/hamstring flexibility	Seated wide-legged forward bend (page 38)	1	2–3 minutes	None
4	Shoulder/chest flexibility	Swimmer's stretch (page 150)	1	1–2 minutes each side	None

HANDSTAND PRACTICE

Exercise	Reps or duration
Set a timer for 5 minutes. Practice walking up into handstand, any variation you like, from pages 40–45. The only rule is that you MUST call it quits after 5 minutes!	5 minutes

TAKING YOUR HANDSTAND OFF THE WALL: **DAY 2**

WARM-UP				
Spend a few breaths moving in downward-facing dog (walking in place, etc.) + follow with a few wrist stretches. (These can be the same wrist stretches below in the mobility/stretch portion, or anything else you like!)				
DRILLS, HIIT-STYLE 4 sets total, alternating exercises A through D (like a circuit). Alternate 30 seconds of work, 10 seconds of rest.				
	Purpose	Exercise	Sets	Reps or duration	Rest
A	Build momentum/ endurance	Side-to-side downward-facing-dog jumps (page 32)	4	30 seconds	10 seconds
B	Upper body strength/ endurance	30-second plank or forearm plank hold	4	30 seconds	10 seconds
C	Hip/lower-body mobility, endurance	Lizard-lunge switches (page 34)	4	30 seconds	10 seconds
D	Overall control/balance + hip mobility	Downward-facing-dog hop switches (page 86)	4	30 seconds	10 seconds

MOBILITY + FLEXIBILITY WORK				
	Purpose	Exercise	Sets	Reps or duration	Rest
1	Wrist relief	Choose 1–2 from the list on page 92	1	1–2 minutes each/each side	None
2	Hip/calf/ankle mobility	Garland pose (squat, page 39)	1	1 minute	None
3	Hamstring flexibility	Seated forward fold (page 152)	1	1-2 minutes	None

HANDSTAND PRACTICE	
Exercise	Reps or duration
Set a timer for 5 minutes. Practice either of the handstand "hoptions" on pages 46–49. Rest as needed in between tries + do both sides. Start near a wall + gradually move away from it as you feel comfortable.	5 minutes

TAKING YOUR HANDSTAND OFF THE WALL: DAY 3

		WARM-UP			
		Spend a few breaths moving in downward-facing dog (walking in place, etc.) + follow with a few wrist stretches. (These can be the same wrist stretches below in the mobility/stretch portion, or anything else you like!)			
		DRILLS, HIIT-STYLE 4 sets total, alternating exercises A through D (like a circuit). Alternate 30 seconds of work, 10 seconds of rest.			
	Purpose	Exercise	Sets	Reps or duration	Rest
A	Hip/lower-body mobility, endurance	Lizard-lunge switches (page 34)	4	30 seconds	10 seconds
B	Shoulder/upper-body strength + stability	Transition back + forth between plank, side plank on left, plank, side plank on right	4	30 seconds	10 seconds
C	Endurance, momentum, hip mobility	Yoga burpees (page 30)	4	30 seconds	10 seconds
D	Overall control/balance + hip mobility	Downward- facing-dog hop switches (page 86)	1	30 seconds	10 seconds

MOBILITY + FLEXIBILITY WORK

	Purpose	Exercise	Sets	Reps or duration	Rest
1	Wrist relief	Choose 1–2 from the list on page 92	1	1–2 minutes each/each side	None
2	Hip/calf/ankle mobility	Garland pose (squat, page 39)	1	1 minute	None
3	Shoulder + hamstring flexibility	Standing wide-legged forward fold with hand clasp or strap (page 149)	1	1 minute	None

HANDSTAND PRACTICE

Exercise	Reps or duration
Set timer for 5 minutes. Practice either handstand hops or jumps (pages 46–51) until timer goes off, resting in between tries as needed. Move your mat farther from the wall over time.	5 minutes

LEARNING FOREARM STAND: DAY 1

WARM-UP
Spend a few breaths moving in downward-facing dog as you like. Then do 4 rounds of downward-facing dog to dolphin to forearm plank: Begin in downward-facing dog with hands turned out slightly, focus on hugging elbows in as you lower. Let elbows hover for a count of 5 before lowering all the way down to dolphin. Stay a few breaths, then walk feet back to forearm plank. Stay for a few breaths, then walk up into plank (alternate lead hands each set) + press back to downward-facing dog. Do 2–4 rounds.

DRILLS, HIIT-STYLE
3 sets total, alternating exercises A through C (like a circuit).
Alternate 30 seconds of work, 10 seconds of rest.

	Purpose	Exercise	Sets	Reps or duration	Rest
A	Upper-body strength/ core stability, hone shoulder-over-elbow alignment	Plank walks (page 98)	4	30 seconds	10 seconds
B	Lower-body mobility/endurance	Lizard-lunge switches (page 34)	4	30 seconds	10 seconds
C	Shoulder + core strength/stability, balance	Forearm side plank (page 101)	4 total (2 on each side)	30 seconds each side; switch sides each round	10 seconds

MOBILITY + FLEXIBILITY WORK

	Purpose	Exercise	Sets	Reps or duration	Rest
1	Hip flexibility/mobility	Pigeon (page 36) or firelog pose (page 36)	1	2–3 minutes each/each side	None
2	Quad hip flexor/ ab stretch	Reclined hero pose (page 102)	1	2–3 minutes	None
3	Shoulder, chest + hamstring flexibility	Standing wide-legged forward fold with hand clasp or strap (page 149)	1	1–2 minutes	None
4	Hamstring stretch	Seated forward fold (page 152)	1	1–2 minutes	None

FOREARM STAND PRACTICE

Exercise	Reps or duration
Set a timer for 5 minutes. Practice headless headstand (page 105) at or near the wall, incorporating any props you like. Start with setting up + lifting one leg at a time. If that feels good, try a small hop or a float on each side, perhaps catching some airtime! The only rule is that you MUST call it quits after 5 minutes!	5 minutes

LEARNING FOREARM STAND: DAY 2

WARM-UP
Spend a few breaths moving in downward-facing dog as you like. Then do 4 rounds of downward-facing dog to dolphin to forearm plank: Begin in downward-facing dog with hands turned out slightly, focus on hugging elbows in as you lower. Let elbows hover for a count of 5 before lowering all the way down to dolphin. Stay a few breaths, then walk feet back to forearm plank. Stay for a few breaths, then walk up into plank (alternate lead hands each set) + press back to downward-facing dog. Do 2–4 rounds.

DRILLS, HIIT-STYLE
3 sets total, alternating exercises A through C (like a circuit).
Alternate 30 seconds of work, 10 seconds of rest.

	Purpose	Exercise	Sets	Reps or duration	Rest
A	Upper-body strength + stability	Tricep presses (page 100)	4	30 seconds	10 seconds
B	Lower-body mobility/ endurance	Yoga burpees (page 30)	4	30 seconds	10 seconds
C	Shoulder strength + mobility	Sewing machine drills (page 124)	4	30 seconds	10 seconds

MOBILITY + FLEXIBILITY WORK

	Purpose	Exercise	Sets	Reps or duration	Rest
1	Quad, psoas, chest, + shoulder stretch	Revolved lizard lunge with foot grab (page 103)	1	1 minute each side	None
2	Hip + hamstring flexibility	Yin butterfly with head on block (page 126)	1	1–2 minutes	None
3	Shoulder/chest flexibility	Swimmer's stretch (page 150)	1	1–2 minutes each side	None

FOREARM STAND PRACTICE

Exercise	Reps or duration
Same as day 1. Feel free to try pincha (parallel forearms + gaze forward) in lieu of headless headstand if you'd like!	5 minutes

LEARNING FOREARM STAND: DAY 3

<table>
<tr><th colspan="6" align="center">WARM-UP</th></tr>
<tr><td colspan="6">Spend a few breaths moving in downward-facing dog as you like. Then do 4 rounds of downward-facing dog to dolphin to forearm plank: Begin in downward-facing dog with hands turned out slightly; focus on hugging elbows in as you lower. Let elbows hover for a count of 5 before lowering all the way down to dolphin. Stay a few breaths, then walk feet back to forearm plank. Stay for a few breaths, then walk up into plank (alternate lead hands each set) + press back to downward-facing dog. Do 2–4 rounds.</td></tr>
<tr><td colspan="6" align="center">DRILLS, HIIT-STYLE
3 sets total, alternating exercises A through C (like a circuit).
Alternate 30 seconds of work, 10 seconds of rest.</td></tr>
<tr><td></td><td>Purpose</td><td>Exercise</td><td>Sets</td><td>Reps or duration</td><td>Rest</td></tr>
<tr><td>A</td><td>Upper-body strength + stability, hone shoulder-over-elbow alignment</td><td>Forearm plank</td><td>4</td><td>30 seconds</td><td>10 seconds</td></tr>
<tr><td>B</td><td>Hip mobility/ endurance</td><td>Your choice! Lizard-lunge switches (page 34) or yoga burpees (page 30)</td><td>4</td><td>30 seconds</td><td>10 seconds</td></tr>
<tr><td>C</td><td>Shoulder strength + mobility, hone elbow-over-shoulder alignment</td><td>Forearm side plank (page 101). Start with 2 on each side + throughout the month, try to gradually work up to 8 rounds on each side.</td><td>4–8 (2–4 each side, then switch sides)</td><td>30 seconds</td><td>10 seconds</td></tr>
</table>

MOBILITY + STATIC STRETCHING

	Purpose	Exercise	Sets	Reps or duration	Rest
1	Mild backbend, hamstring stretch	Inverted action pose with block under pelvis (page 156)	1	1–2 minutes	None
2	Psoas, quad, chest + shoulder stretch	Hip-flexor stretch on block (page 104)	1	1–2 minutes (both legs at once) or 1 minute each side	None
3	Shoulder/ upper-back stretch	Puppy pose (page 127)	1	1–2 minutes	None

FOREARM STAND PRACTICE

Exercise	Reps or duration
Same as day 2.	5 minutes

BLANK PRACTICE GRID: DAY 1

WARM-UP				
DRILLS, HIIT-STYLE 4 sets total, alternating exercises A through D (like a circuit). Alternate 30 seconds of work, 10 seconds of rest.				
	Purpose	Exercise	Sets	Reps or duration	Rest
A					
B					
C					
D					

MOBILITY + FLEXIBILITY WORK

	Purpose	Exercise	Sets	Reps or duration	Rest
1					
2					
3					

INVERSION PRACTICE

Exercise	Reps or duration

BLANK PRACTICE GRID: DAY 2

WARM-UP				

DRILLS, HIIT-STYLE 4 sets total, alternating exercises A through D (like a circuit). Alternate 30 seconds of work, 10 seconds of rest.				
	Purpose	Exercise	Sets	Reps or duration	Rest
A					
B					
C					
D					

MOBILITY + FLEXIBILITY WORK

	Purpose	Exercise	Sets	Reps or duration	Rest
1					
2					
3					

INVERSION PRACTICE

Exercise	Reps or duration

BLANK PRACTICE GRID: DAY 3

WARM-UP

DRILLS, HIIT-STYLE
4 sets total, alternating exercises A through D (like a circuit).
Alternate 30 seconds of work, 10 seconds of rest.

	Purpose	Exercise	Sets	Reps or duration	Rest
A					
B					
C					
D					

MOBILITY + FLEXIBILITY WORK

	Purpose	Exercise	Sets	Reps or duration	Rest
1					
2					
3					

INVERSION PRACTICE

Exercise	Reps or duration

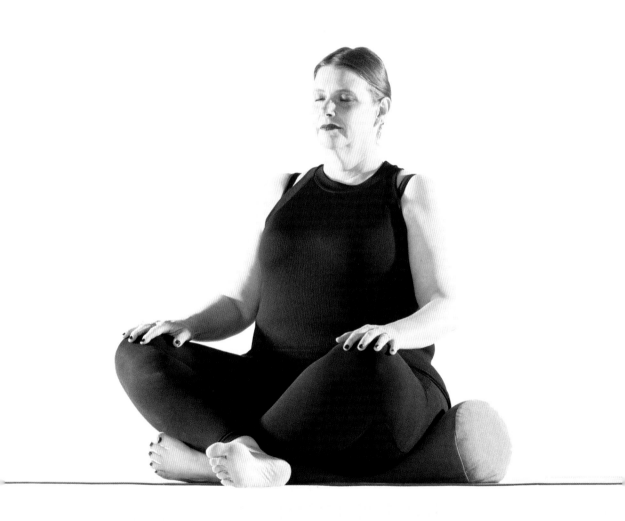

Appendix 2

Sample Yoga Sequence Blueprint

You may recall a similar sequence blueprint if you've read *Yoga Where You Are*. And as Dianne and I explained in that book, there are many ways to sequence a yoga practice. This is just one example, but it can be a great starting place for planning out a practice.

If you use this blueprint, you don't have to do a pose for every category. Skip any that don't fit with your present needs, goals, or intentions for practice.

CENTERING: A simple and comfortable sitting, kneeling, standing, or lying pose with a simple reflection and breath-awareness work.

WARM-UP: Simple, dynamic movements, preparatory stages of poses—for example, a low lunge if you're going to be doing a high lunge later.

DOWNWARD-FACING DOG: Include dynamic movements to start, such as pedaling the feet, shifting hips and heels from side to side. Introduce options and alternatives, like bending the knees, placing hands on blocks, coming to forearms for dolphin, or coming to hands and knees or puppy pose.

SUN SALUTATIONS: Any variation that you like.

STANDING POSES: Warrior poses, standing balance poses, lunge variations, and so on.

CORE WORK: Planks, hollow-hold variations, exercises borrowed from other styles of movement such as Pilates.

HIP OPENERS: Think poses like forward-bend variations of pigeon, firelog, lizard lunge, and more.

ARM BALANCES AND ACTIVE/ARM-BALANCING INVERSIONS: This is the place for hand- and arm-balancing poses like crow, and also for hand- and arm-balancing inversions and/or specific preps and drills for them, including handstand and forearm stand. I also like to sequence headstand here because of its similarity to shoulderstand and the amount of strength, focus, and balance it takes to do. I want to make sure I get to it before I'm too tired!

QUAD AND HIP-FLEXOR STRETCHES: Reclined hero pose, revolved lizard lunge with a foot grab, block-supported hip-flexor stretches, and the like. These help prepare for the backbends that follow, which require a fair amount of quad and hip-flexor flexibility. But if you're practicing inversions that incorporate a backbend, such as pincha mayurasana, hollowback, or scorpion pose, you might prefer to practice at least a few of these beforehand.

BACKBENDS: Bridge pose, wheel pose, bow pose, and more.

SEATED TWISTS AND FORWARD FOLDS: Think seated twists, seated forward bend (paschimottanasana), yin butterfly, seated wide-legged forward bend: poses that help you start to wind down and move inward.

INVERSIONS CONSIDERED MORE MEDITATIVE, RESTORATIVE, OR INWARD MOVING: These are typically the inversions that you may hold for a longer period of time, but you may also find shorter holds to be more appropriate. There's no time minimum or requirement. These poses are also often said to prepare us for relaxation, meditation, and pranayama, which, along with the fact that some of them require a lot of preparation, is why they're often sequenced near the end of class. They include:

- Legs-up-the-wall variations

- Inverted action pose variations

- Shoulderstand variations

- Plow variations

COUNTER POSES FOR SHOULDERSTAND AND PLOW: Restorative fish pose, a supine (lying) butterfly pose, legs-over-a-chair pose. There are also folks who find that gentle prone (belly down) backbends such as cobra or locust (commonly called "superhero pose" in other movement modalities) are helpful counters for shoulderstand, as they bring your neck and shoulders into a direction opposite of what gravity tends to move us toward in shoulderstand.

SUPINE (LYING DOWN) TWISTS AND FORWARD BENDS: Gentle twists, simple knees-to-chest variations, happy baby pose. Any final "feel good" stretches and movements to prepare you for savasana.

SAVASANA: Savasana is most commonly done and depicted lying supine, but you can use this time to do any pose that feels relaxing to you, where you don't have to put in much or any effort to maintain it, such as child's pose, a comfortable seated position, lying on your side, or lying on your belly. You can also do a restorative pose such as legs up the wall here.

PRANAYAMA AND MEDITATION: This could be a guided practice or simply a few moments of silence for breath awareness and reflection.

Resources

(a.k.a. Books Mentioned in This Book)

Embrace Yoga's Roots: Courageous Ways to Deepen Your Yoga Practice
by Susanna Barkataki

Original Yoga: Rediscovering Traditional Practices of Hatha Yoga
by Richard Rosen

The Power of Ashtanga Yoga and *The Power of Ashtanga Yoga II*
by Kino MacGregor

Yoga Biomechanics: Stretching Redefined
by Jules Mitchell

Yoga Where You Are: Customize Your Practice for Your Body and Your Life
by Dianne Bondy and Kat Heagberg

Your Body, Your Yoga
by Bernie Clark

Meet the Models

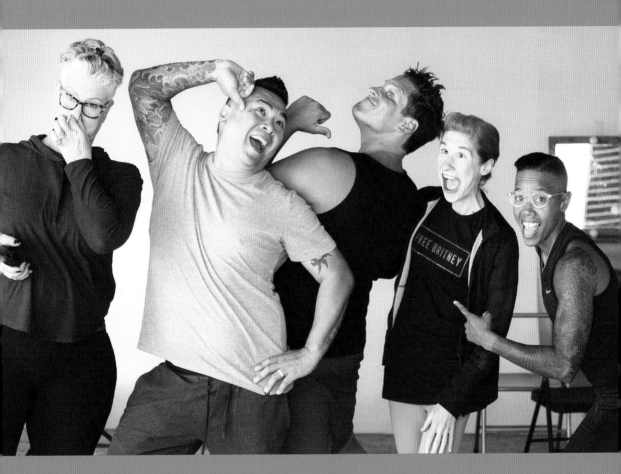

KAT HEAGBERG REBAR (She/Her/They/Them)

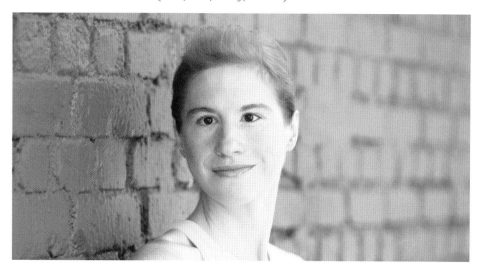

TELL US A LITTLE BIT ABOUT YOU: I started teaching yoga in college and have been at it ever since. These days, I most enjoy teaching "outside of the box" vinyasa classes: unconventional flows in unconventional spaces for "yoga weirdos" like me—those who feel more comfortable in a bar or an art gallery (or a bar that is also an art gallery!) than a typical studio. I'm also a runner and cyclist, and I enjoy teaching cross-training and recovery-focused classes for athletes. I live in Santa Monica, California, with my husband and fellow model Kyle, and in addition to hosting weird yoga events together in our spare time, we also host weird improv comedy shows!

WHAT'S YOUR FAVORITE INVERSION? Hands down (literally), it's handstand!

WHAT'S YOUR CURRENT INVERSION GOAL OR SOMETHING YOU'RE WORKING ON? I'm working on doing a handstand press with my hands elevated on blocks, which increases the load and requires more strength. I also want to learn to walk on my hands because my friend's daughter told me that would be very impressive.

WHAT'S YOUR FAVORITE TYPE OF YOGA OR MOVEMENT PRACTICE? Anything that keeps my brain busy along with my body, like vinyasa flows with interesting choreography and sequencing, or that gets my heart rate up, like yoga/HIIT fusion classes.

WHAT'S A FUN FACT ABOUT YOU? I absolutely love the Muppets. Cookie Monster is my favorite.

KYLE REBAR (He/Him)

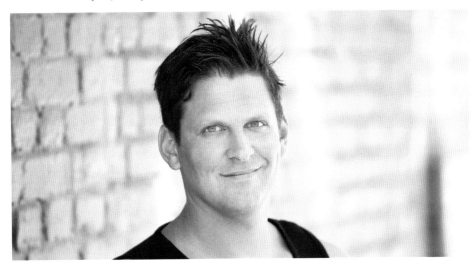

TELL US A LITTLE BIT ABOUT YOU: I'm a Scranton, Pennsylvania, to Santa Monica, California, transplant who loves bass guitars, beach cleanups, improv, and surfing.

YOUR FAVORITE INVERSION: Shoulderstand! It's the one inversion I can easily pull off during performance-art night at open mics. The crowd expects a crooner and they get shoulderstands: always a hit!

WHAT'S YOUR CURRENT INVERSION GOAL OR SOMETHING YOU'RE WORKING ON? I've been working toward a full-range handstand push-up at the wall. Recently while surfing, I saw someone pop up into a tripod headstand on their longboard while riding a wave in—I'd love to do that someday too.

WHAT'S YOUR FAVORITE TYPE OF YOGA OR MOVEMENT PRACTICE? I think yoga is a dish served best in an art gallery with live music. I mostly do yin yoga for mobility on recovery days. My main movement loves these days are CrossFit, Olympic weightlifting, and surfing. I'll also take my kettlebells for long walks sometimes too.

WHAT'S A FUN FACT ABOUT YOU? I've been taking photographs of trash I find on walks since 2017. When I moved to Santa Monica, I started volunteering for beach cleanups and that led me to study environmental science at the local community college. I never thought I'd move to Los Angeles and get into science, but here we are—life's an adventure!

NAM CHANTERWYN (He/Him/His)

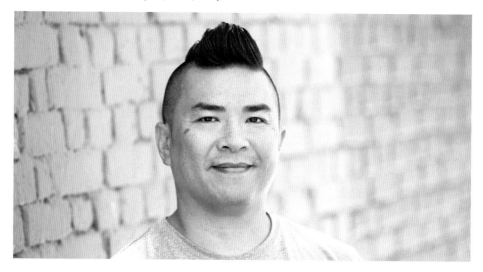

TELL US A LITTLE BIT ABOUT YOU: My lifelong goal is to learn to operate every major vehicle on land, sea, and air. I've already accomplished: land (motorcycle, car, semitruck) and sea (sailboat and speedboat). I've yet to accomplish air (fly a plane and a helicopter). I should have the plane checked off my list by the time this book comes out.

WHAT'S YOUR FAVORITE INVERSION? Handstands are my favorite.

WHAT'S YOUR CURRENT INVERSION GOAL OR SOMETHING YOU'RE WORKING ON? My current goal is finding more core awareness and space in my back body, enabling me to drop my head in handstands and create more length.

WHAT'S YOUR FAVORITE TYPE OF YOGA OR MOVEMENT PRACTICE? I love movement in general and try to vary my movement practice as much as possible, so it's hard to choose a favorite. I find that it's important to find diverse movement practices because no one type will provide everything you need. There are always biases and missing elements in any one movement practice.

WHAT'S A FUN FACT ABOUT YOU? I have a really hard time saying the word *snickerdoodle*. It takes an incredible amount of patience and concentration for me to pronounce the word with proper annunciation.

PEGGY GARTIN (She/Her)

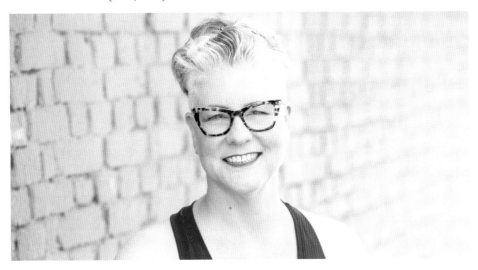

TELL US A LITTLE BIT ABOUT YOU: I'm a web content designer from San Diego, California, who has been practicing yoga for about six years. I started practicing at age fifty as a way to address back pain. Now I practice daily and enjoy the mobility, flexibility, and endurance it brings. My advice: anyone can do yoga! I told myself for years that I wasn't athletic or that, as a bigger person, physical challenges weren't for me. I was so wrong. When I got out of my own way and tried it, I found yoga was a way to honor my body and thank it for all it does for me. And it can do more than I thought. My first headstand blew my mind!

WHAT'S YOUR FAVORITE INVERSION? My favorite inversion is your everyday downward-facing dog, but I also enjoy standing wide-legged forward fold.

WHAT'S YOUR CURRENT INVERSION GOAL OR SOMETHING YOU'RE WORKING ON? Getting the top of my head to touch the floor in that forward fold.

WHAT'S YOUR FAVORITE TYPE OF YOGA OR MOVEMENT PRACTICE? Vinyasa flow or stick mobility practices.

WHAT'S A FUN FACT ABOUT YOU? My husband and I are restoring our 120-year-old house, and the hardwood floors are perfect for going upside down.

SARAH TACOMA (She/Her)

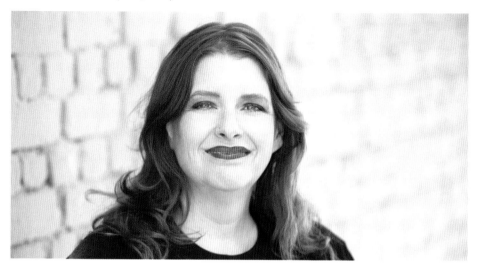

TELL US A LITTLE BIT ABOUT YOU: I'm a stay-at-home and work-from-home mom of two teenage boys. I'm a freelance graphic designer who enjoys card playing, decorating, and hiking.

WHAT'S YOUR FAVORITE INVERSION? Downward-facing dog at the wall.

WHAT'S YOUR CURRENT INVERSION GOAL OR SOMETHING YOU'RE WORKING ON? Finding ways to incorporate yoga into my daily life and exercise routines.

WHAT'S YOUR FAVORITE TYPE OF YOGA OR MOVEMENT PRACTICE? Hiking, dancing, and boot-camp classes.

WHAT'S A FUN FACT ABOUT YOU? I'm an obsessive thrift-store shopper.

DR. C. SHANTÉ COFIELD, a.k.a. THE MAESTRO (She/Her/They/Them)

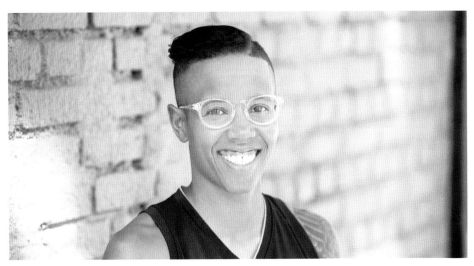

TELL US A LITTLE BIT ABOUT YOU: I'm a physical therapist turned entrepreneur. I host the podcast *Maestro on the Mic*, and I'm the founder of The Movement Maestro LLC, a social media–based company that provides both online and in-person education for health and movement professionals around the world. My professional pursuits center around providing business coaching, with a focus on brand strategy and community development in the ever-growing digital marketplace. I'm also a proud SoCal resident, I drive a hypergreen Jeep Wrangler, and I wish to leave you with this message: be relentless in the pursuit of what sets your soul on fire.

WHAT'S YOUR FAVORITE INVERSION? Freestanding handstand.

WHAT'S YOUR CURRENT INVERSION GOAL OR SOMETHING YOU'RE WORKING ON? My fitness pursuits (beach volleyball) don't have me working on a lot of inversions these days, but it's always fun to revisit handstands and handstand walking to make sure I still got it.

WHAT'S YOUR FAVORITE TYPE OF YOGA OR MOVEMENT PRACTICE? I'm absolutely a yoga muggle, and my preference is hot yoga if I'm gonna practice. As for my preferred movement practices, I'm obsessed with beach volleyball, and my garage gym is absolutely my happy place.

WHAT'S A FUN FACT ABOUT YOU? My cat, Rupert the Meowstro, is my best friend, and he has definitely made me a better person.

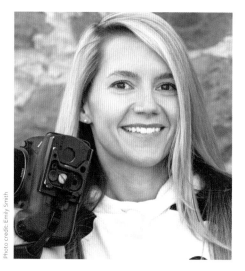

Photo credit: Emily Smith

TELL US A LITTLE BIT ABOUT YOU: I've been a photographer since 1995 and started my business in 2008. My goal has always been to help individuals and brands tell their stories through authentic, powerful images, and my areas of focus include interiors, food, and lifestyle. I was photographer and creative director for Yoga International from 2015 to 2021, and I have created a ton of yoga images throughout my career.

WHAT'S YOUR FAVORITE INVERSION? My favorite inversion is forearm stand because of the feeling I had the first time I successfully made it into, and held, the pose.

WHAT'S YOUR CURRENT INVERSION GOAL OR SOMETHING YOU'RE WORKING ON? My dream inversion is press handstand, though whether or not that's physiologically possible for me is to be determined.

WHAT'S YOUR FAVORITE TYPE OF YOGA OR MOVEMENT PRACTICE? My favorite type of movement practice is strength training: squat, deadlift, bench press, overhead press, and rows. I lift three times per week, and I walk outside every day.

WHAT'S A FUN FACT ABOUT YOU? I'm a wellness and domestic-life enthusiast. I love cooking fresh, whole foods for family and friends; living in the country; taking care of my small plot of land, garden, twelve chickens, cat, and my loving husband. Low-key farm life has always been my dream, and my family and I are fortunate enough to be living it.